For One Year olds (boys)

Our first Valentine's My Son

A Valentine's

Kids Book for First Moms

to express feelings

A Gift for *him*

ANGELICA ROCKFORD

With love ♡

To my sister Yoni: Congratulations on becoming a mommy for the first time!

It will be amazing experience. Thank you. for giving me a nephew. "I love you."

And another big congratulations to all the new mommys! I send you many blessings and tons of amazing surprises. I love you!

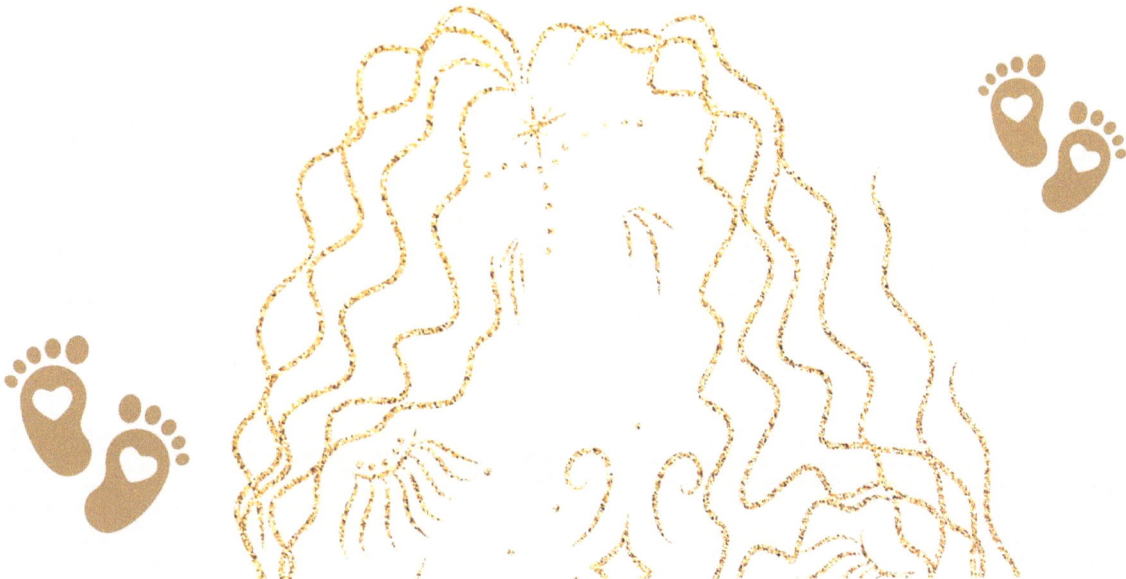

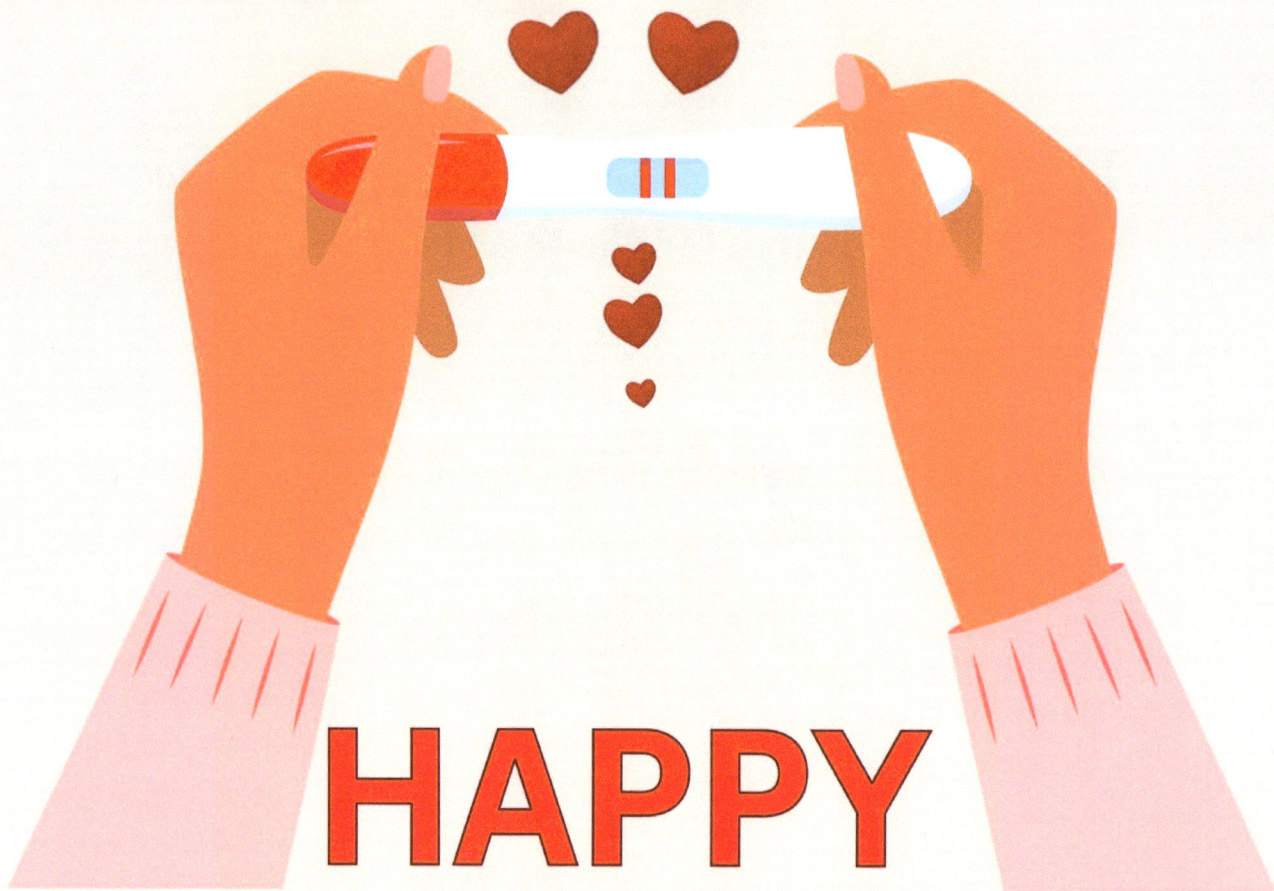

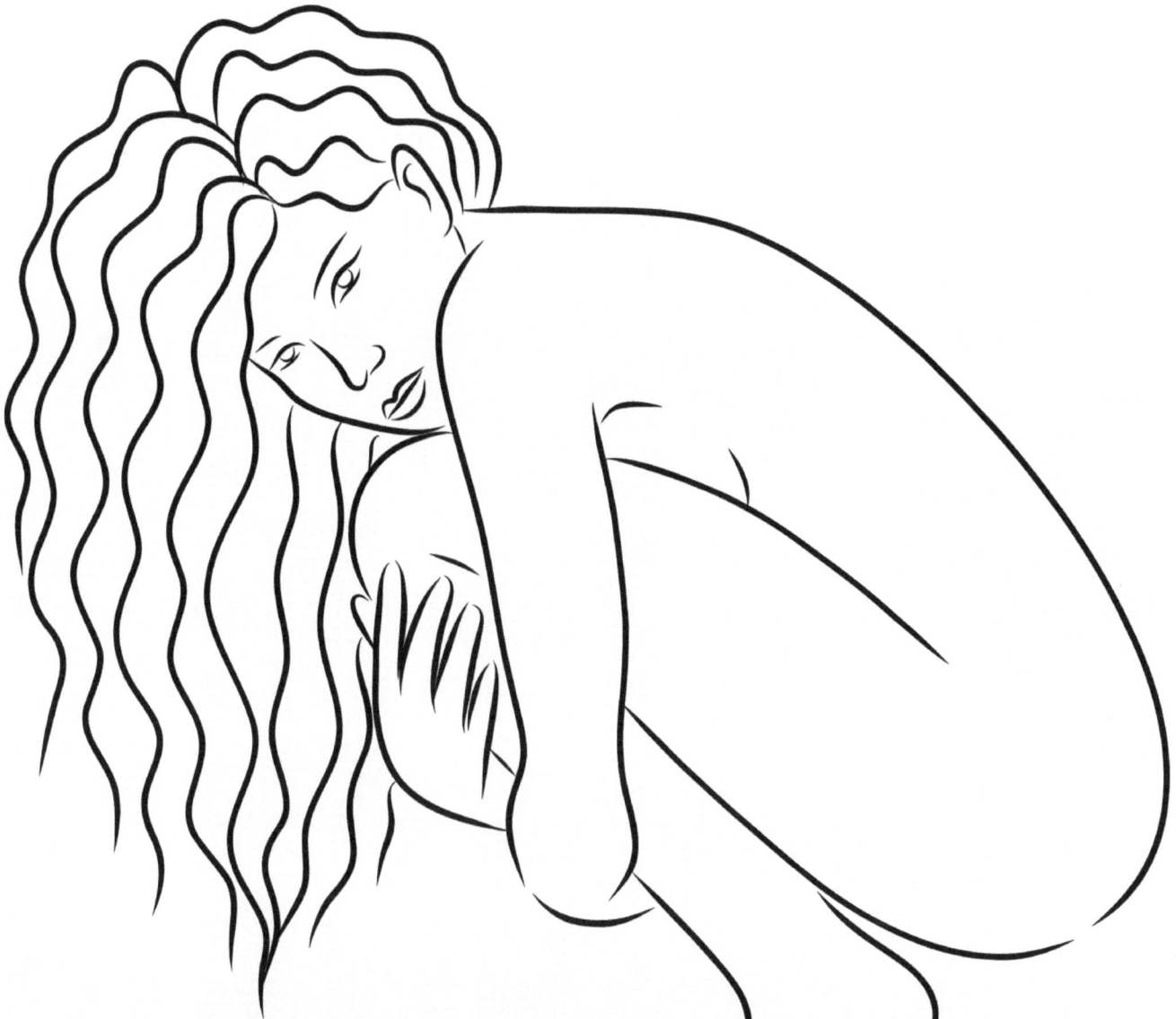

Yes, that is the day when I got pregnant, it was a day like Valentine's Day. And Momma wouldn't lie, she didn't know whether to be happy or scared (actually she was scared.)

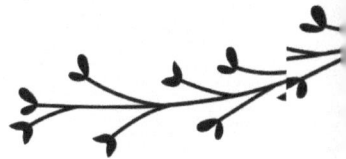

But she decided to be HAPPY, and it happened to be the best decision Momma ever made.

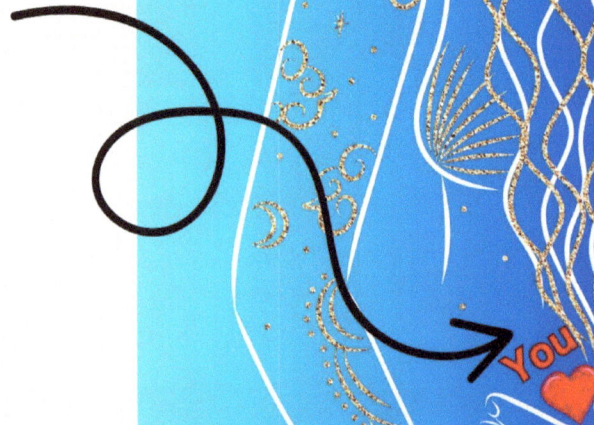

And since then...
I called you my Valentine.

And every day, I've found myself falling more and more in love with being your mommy.

And so time passed...

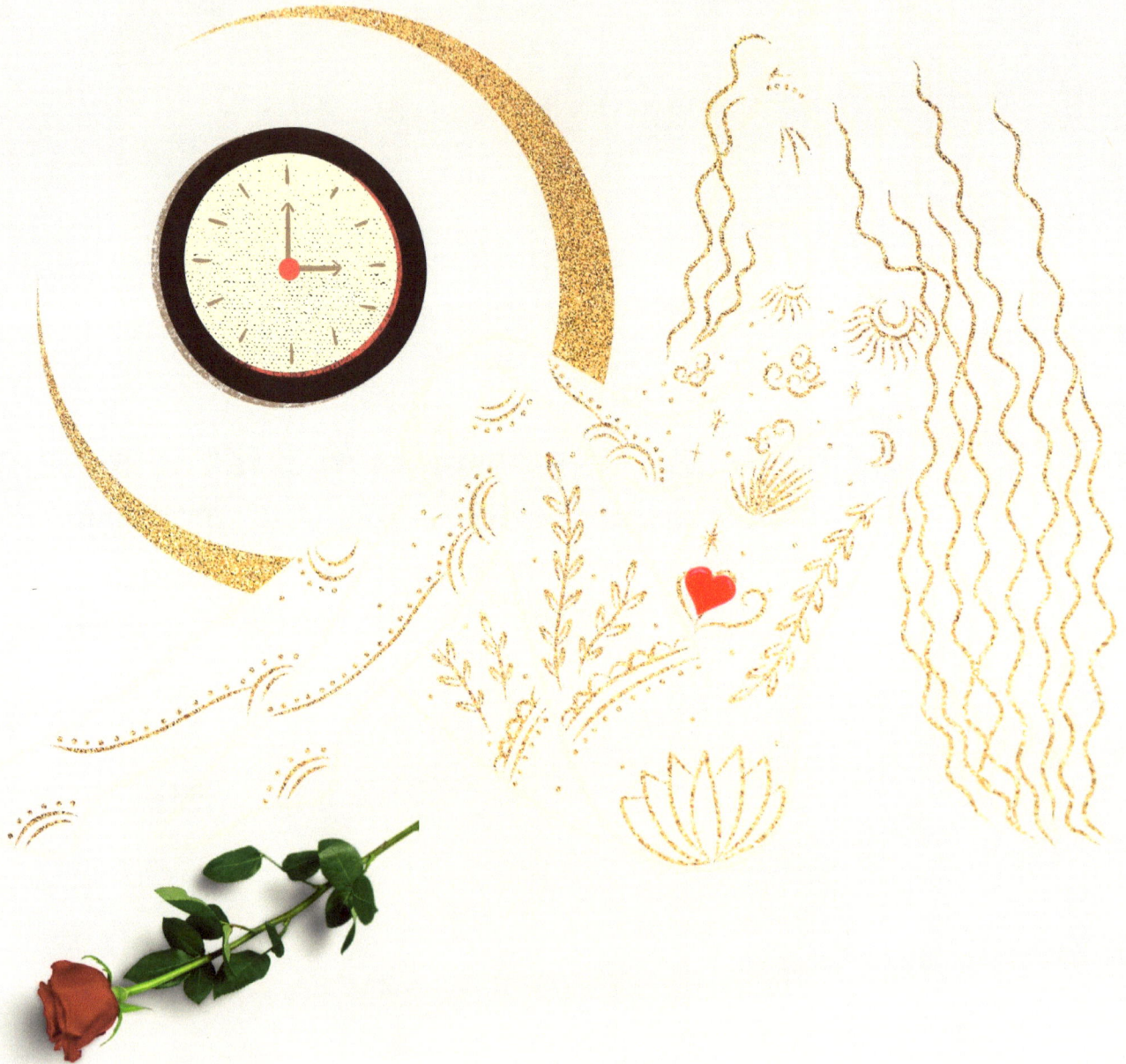

And here I am,
with you in my tummy.
Tumy, tumy, tum, tum.

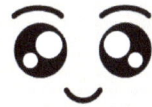

You grow so much!

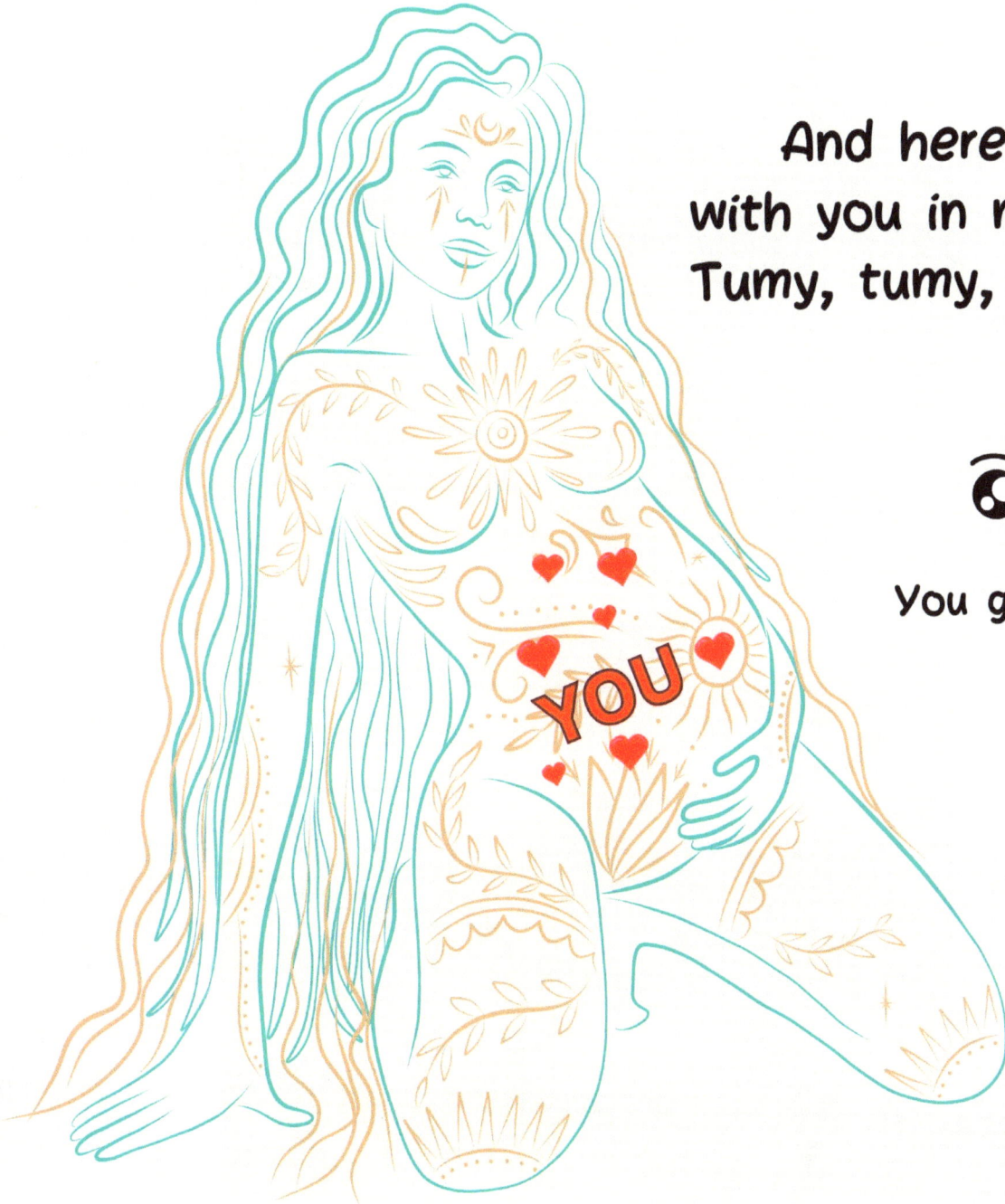

YOU

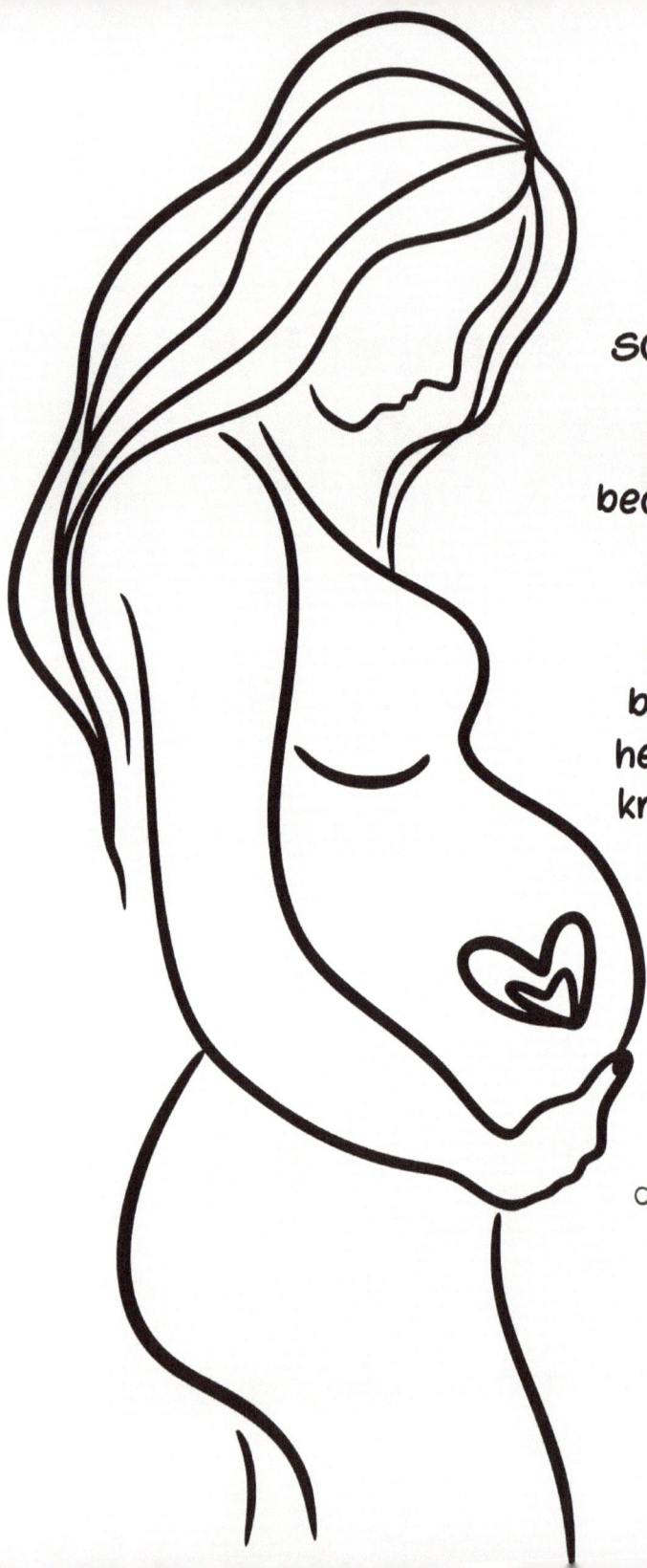

SON, TODAY I WANT TO SING TO YOU.

I want to sing to you without words because tomorrow, we'll meet for the very first time.

With happiness, I sing to you softly; because I feel your heart knows me, it hears me, just as I hear you. Because I know you understand my words, without words, my Valentine, tine, tine, tine.

Today I love you so much.

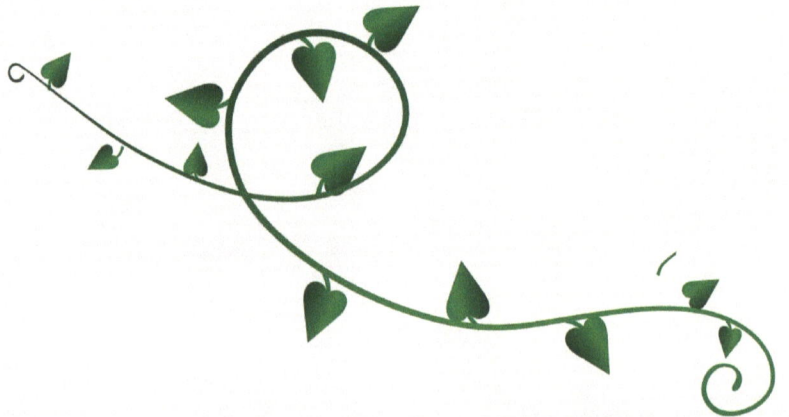

And here you are, so close to me, so close to you,
I welcome you so happily, my darling, it is...

Like your smile, that lights up my life,
Like your eyes, that give me life,
Like your existence, that brought me back to life,
MY Valentine, Valentine, Valentine: You are my
Valentine today, darling...

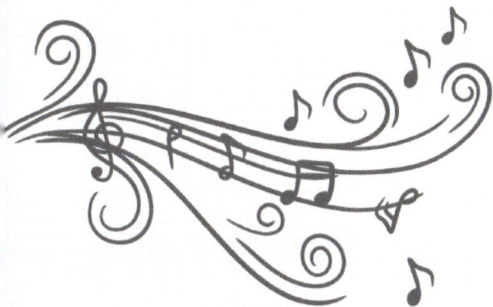

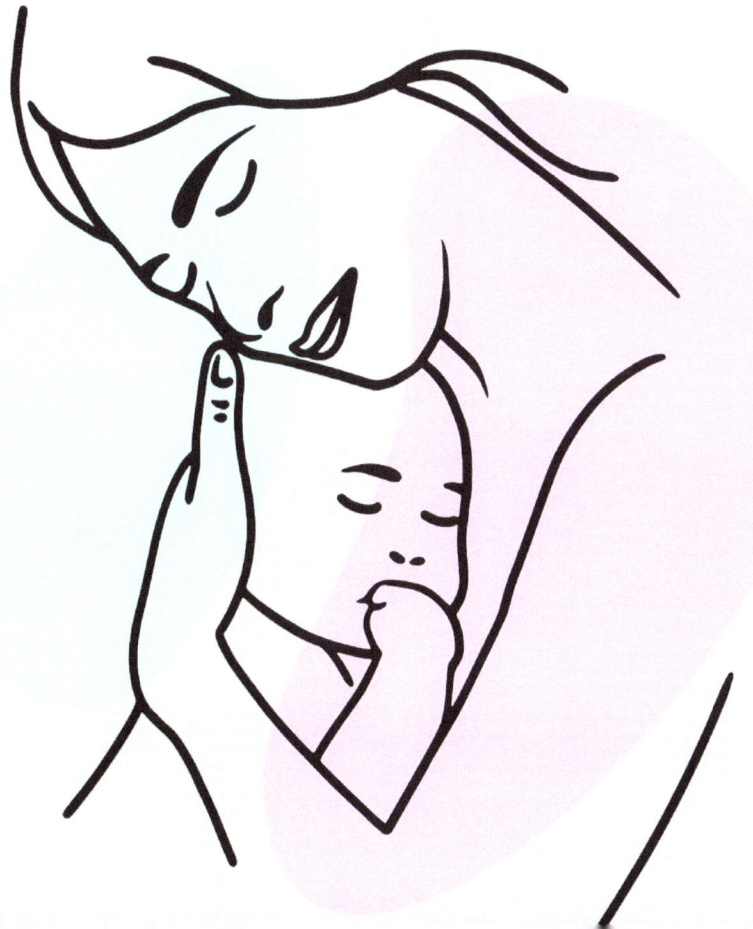

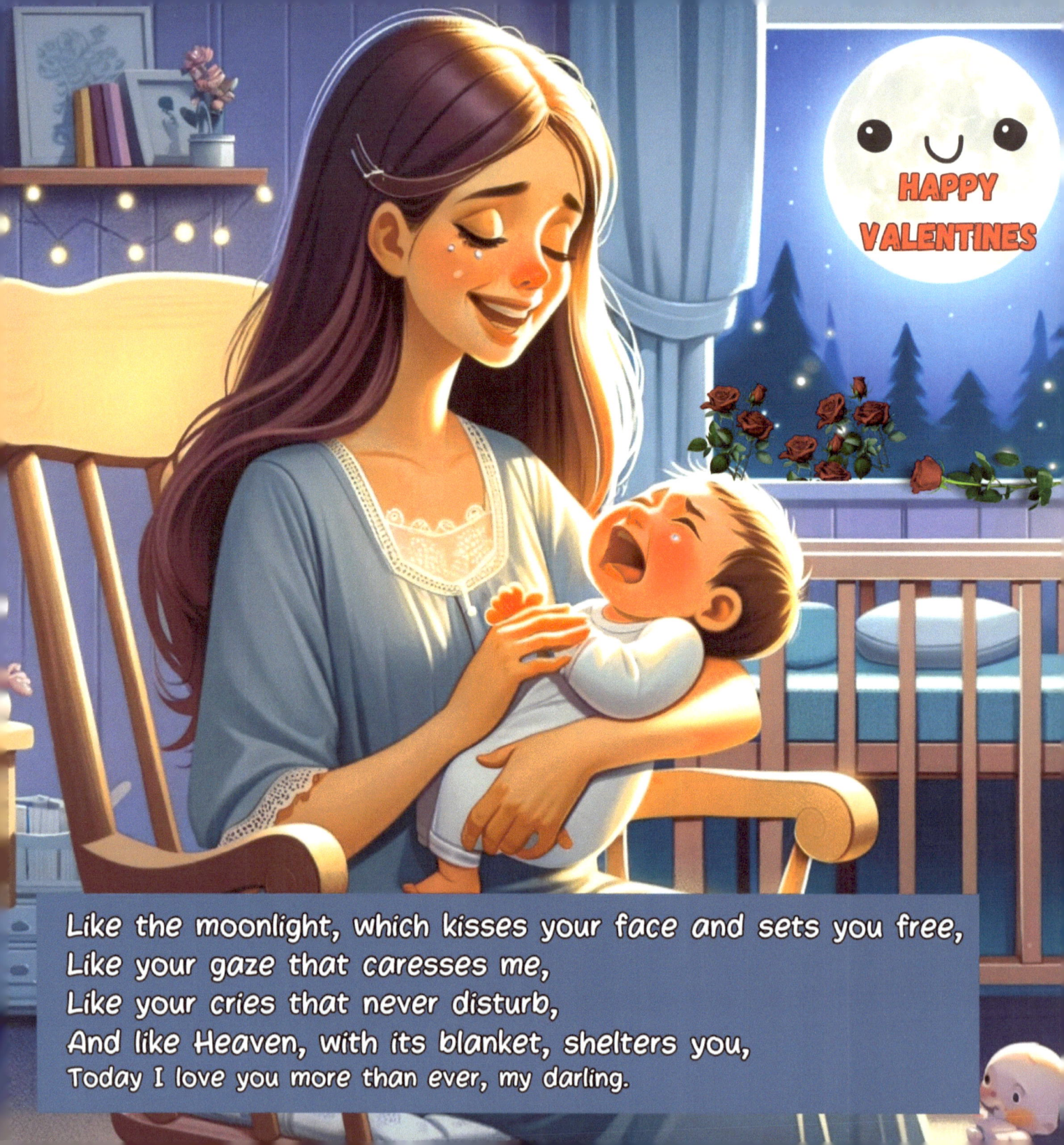

Like the moonlight, which kisses your face and sets you free,
Like your gaze that caresses me,
Like your cries that never disturb,
And like Heaven, with its blanket, shelters you,
Today I love you more than ever, my darling.

As you sleep here in my arms, I sing to you very softly.
You are...
My Christmas,
My Happy New Year,
My VALENTINE, tine, tine, tine, tine,

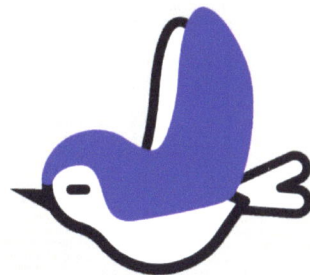

Because with you, every day is my Valentine's,
Today I love you, and I always will, my darling.

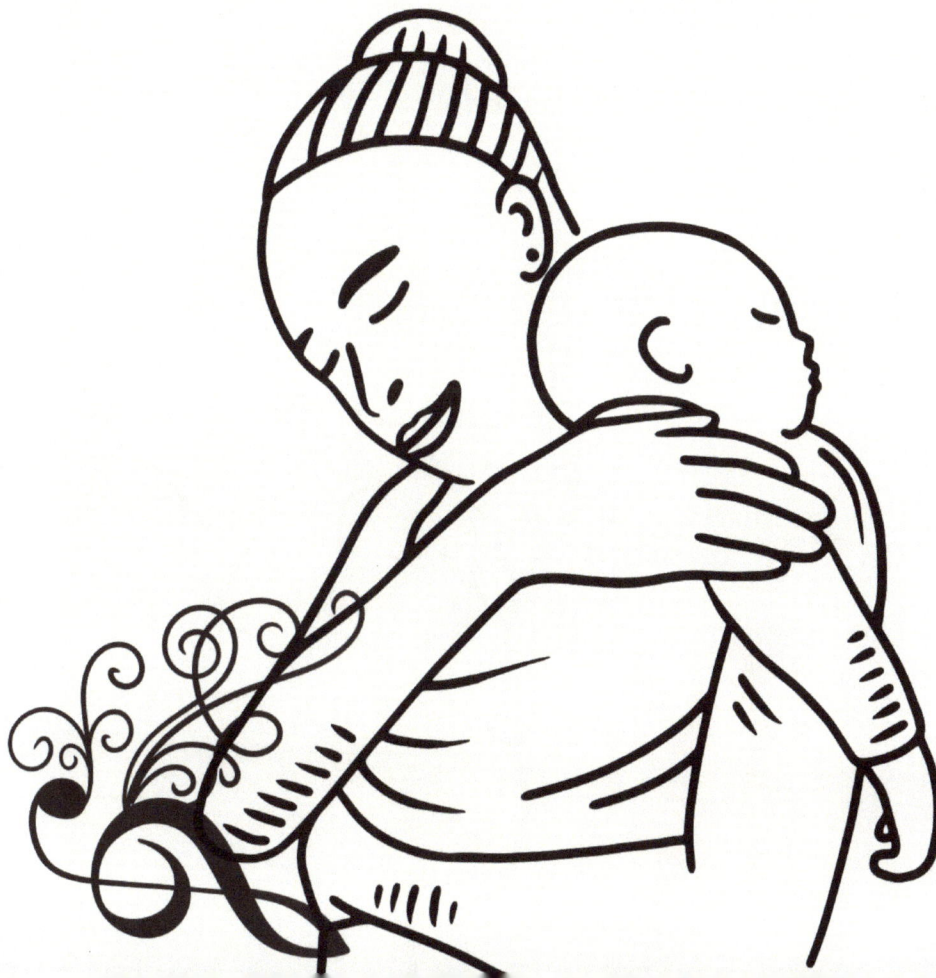

I lovingly hold you in my arms and immediately I melt seeing you sleep for the first time,

I want to do so many things, to teach you all about life, though I know it will be you who will teach me.

My valentine, valentine, valentineeee
You'll always be my Valentine.

Today I love you and always will.

My, baby, bubu, babo.
Momma love you.

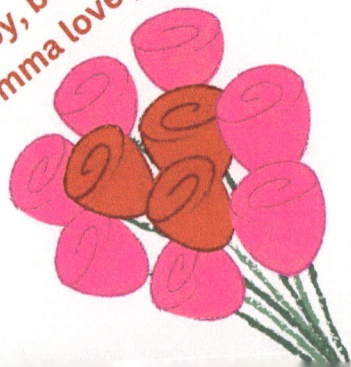

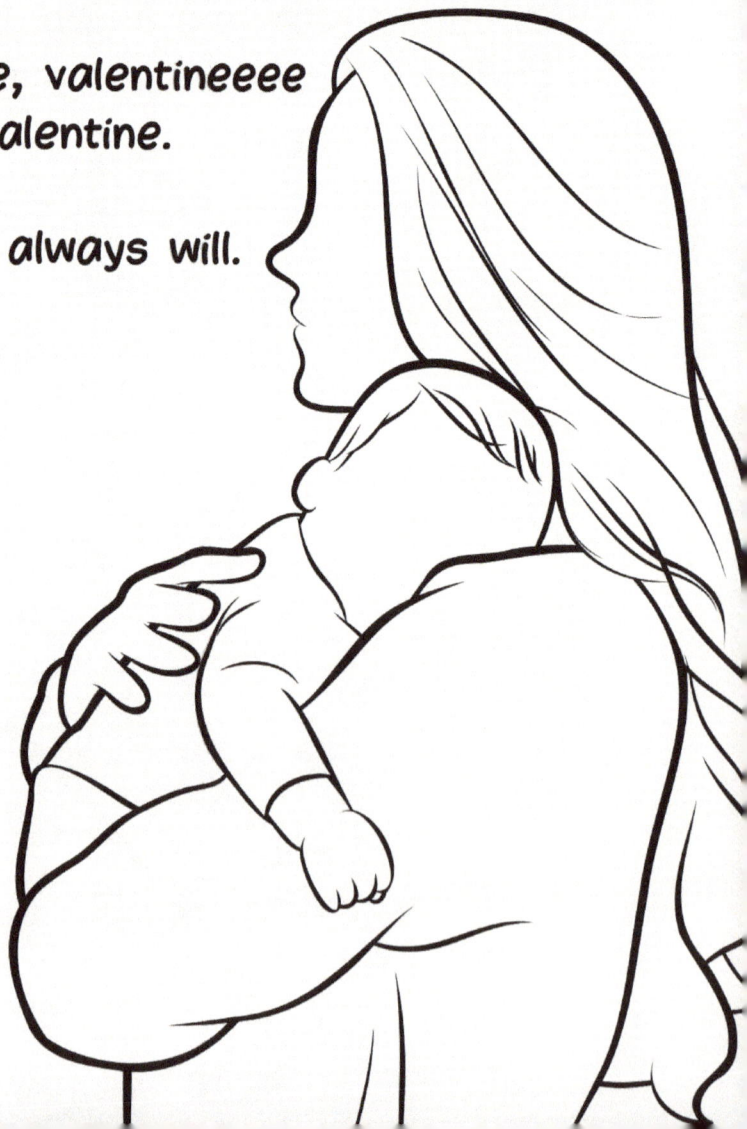

Sleep my baby sleep, because I will sing you the good mornings, and good nights, every day to thank you for being my baby; and no matter what happens, no matter what time gossip. "You will always be my baby," my son I love you today, and always my darling.

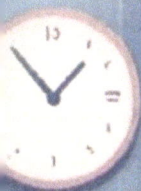

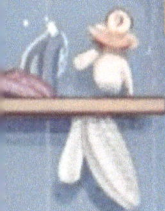

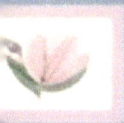

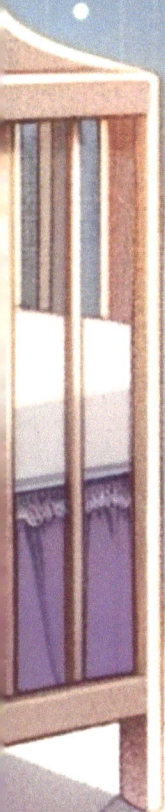

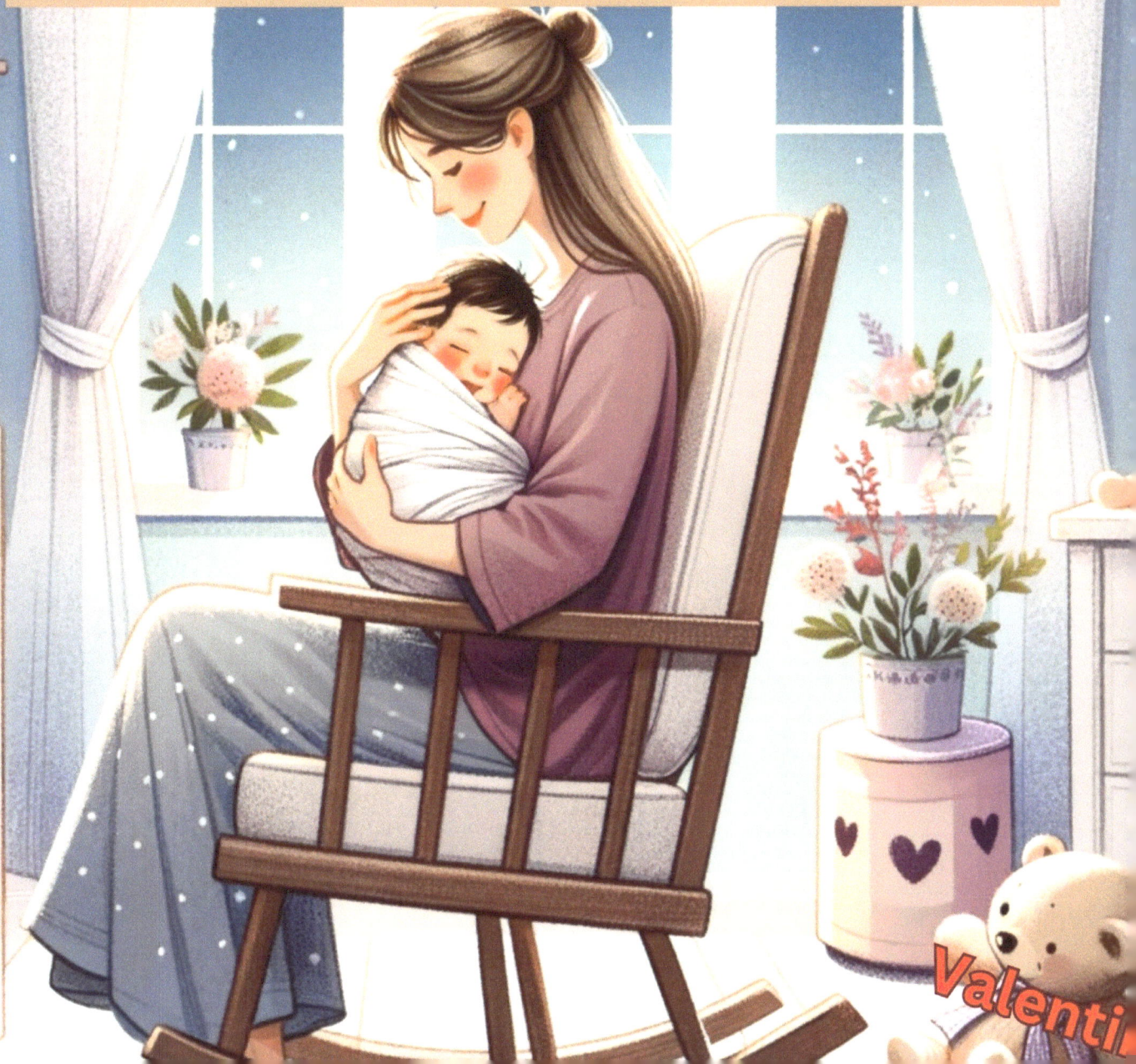

You barely open your eyes and,
 I'm already scared, you'll grow up so fast,
Hay baby, bubu, I love you, I love you,
 I love youuuuuuuuuuuuuuuuuuuu

I will always love you, all my life
I will love you because you are my definition of "love".

Valentine

Just as patience awaits, I can not wait for you to call me 'Momma'
Like the gratitude that thanks you,
Like the life that blesses you, today I love you very much.
Today I am stronger.

....

It feels good being close to you,
It feels like home, my darling,
you are my home,
You are my Valentine, my darling.
You are...

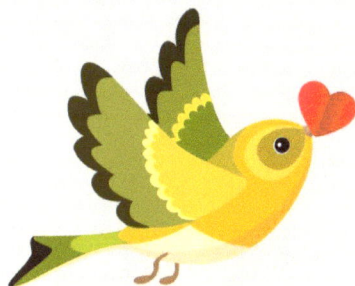

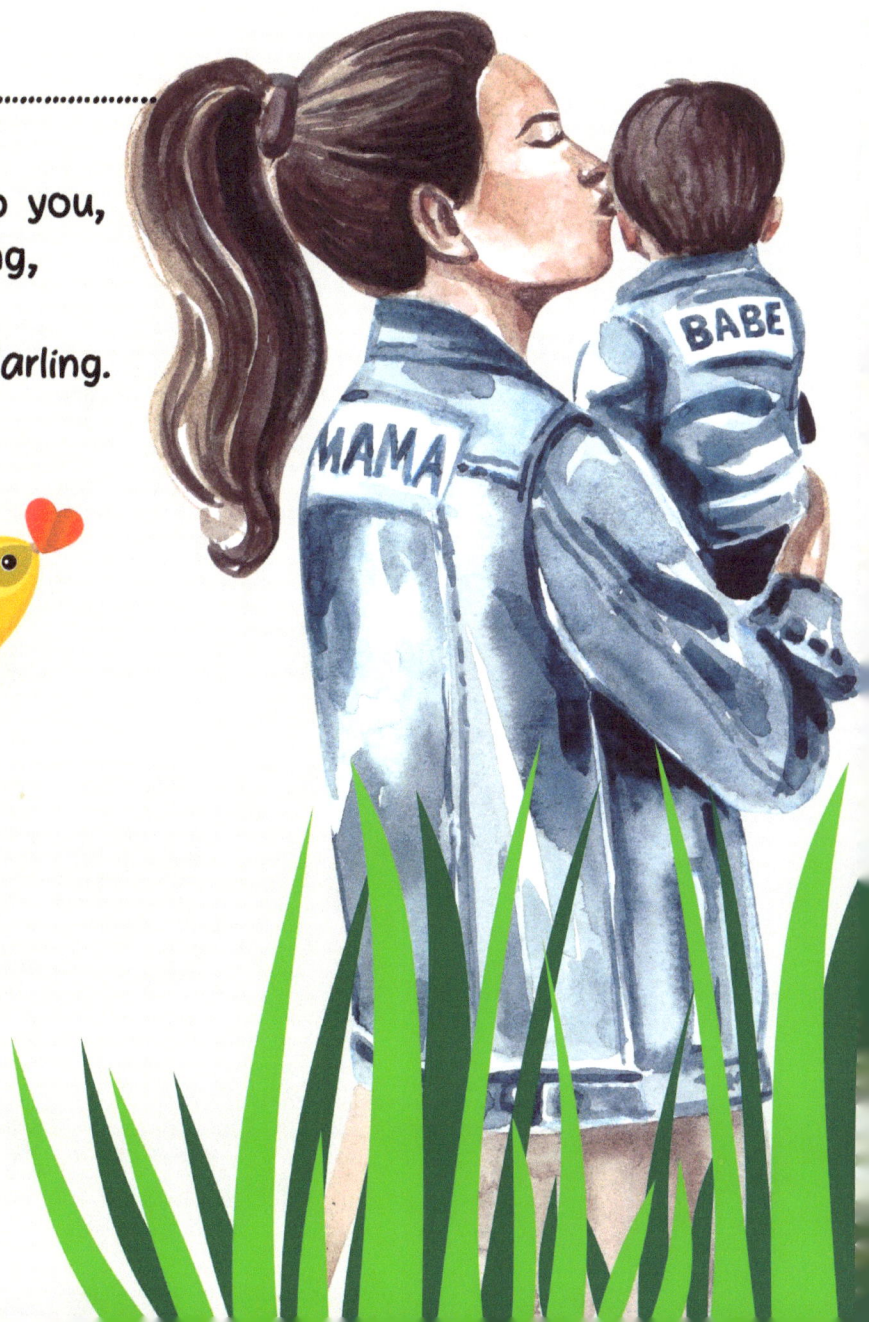

You are what I call Home.

When I am close to you, I feel at home my darling,
you are my home, it always feels good being close
to you.
You are my Valentine, my darling.
You are...

You are what I call Home,
You are the reason why I come back home,
You are the reason I come home,
You are my "home," my darling,

You are my Valentine's home, my baby.
Your soft smile is my Valentine's my bubu.
Today I love you, and always will.
Thank you for being my Valentine's gift.

Momma love you, my bubu, babo.

Today my hands are covered with your love,
Because I know that one day you will grow up, and leave home;
forgive my faltering, in the rush of time, you growing up so fast,
and I... I'm already afraid that it will be tomorrow:

I wish I could stop time, I wish I could stop you.
But I've already understood, that ...I can't.
I resign to tell you,

a piece of my heart will go with you, between your suitcases,
and in the meantime, I will be loving you, strongly.
Today, I love you without fears.

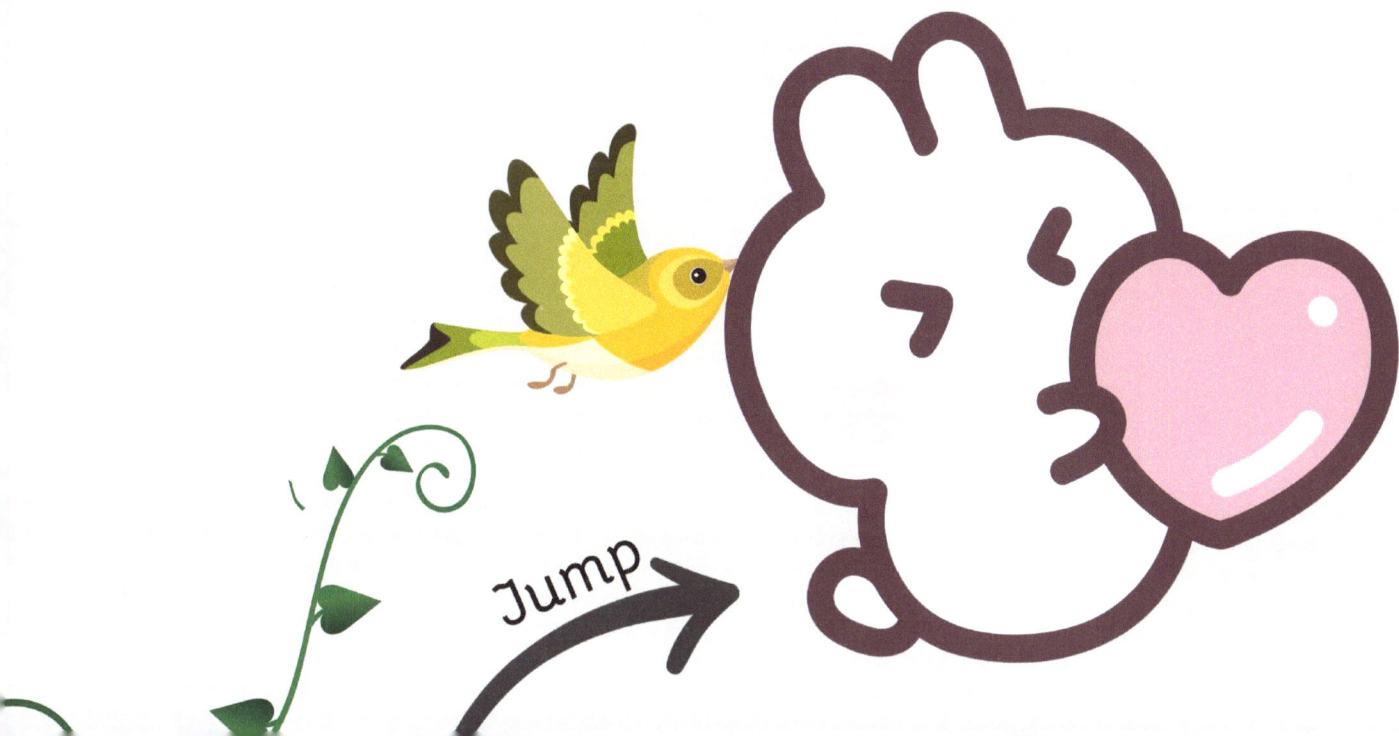

Jump

My valentine, tine, tine,
I will always love you, my Valentine.

....

I will love you without barriers,
I will love you without limits,
I will love you so much, until you
ask me "Why do you love me so
much, Momma".

And I will tell you.... "because you
are simply my son, and I am your
mother;
Because you are my definition of
what I love, my darling.

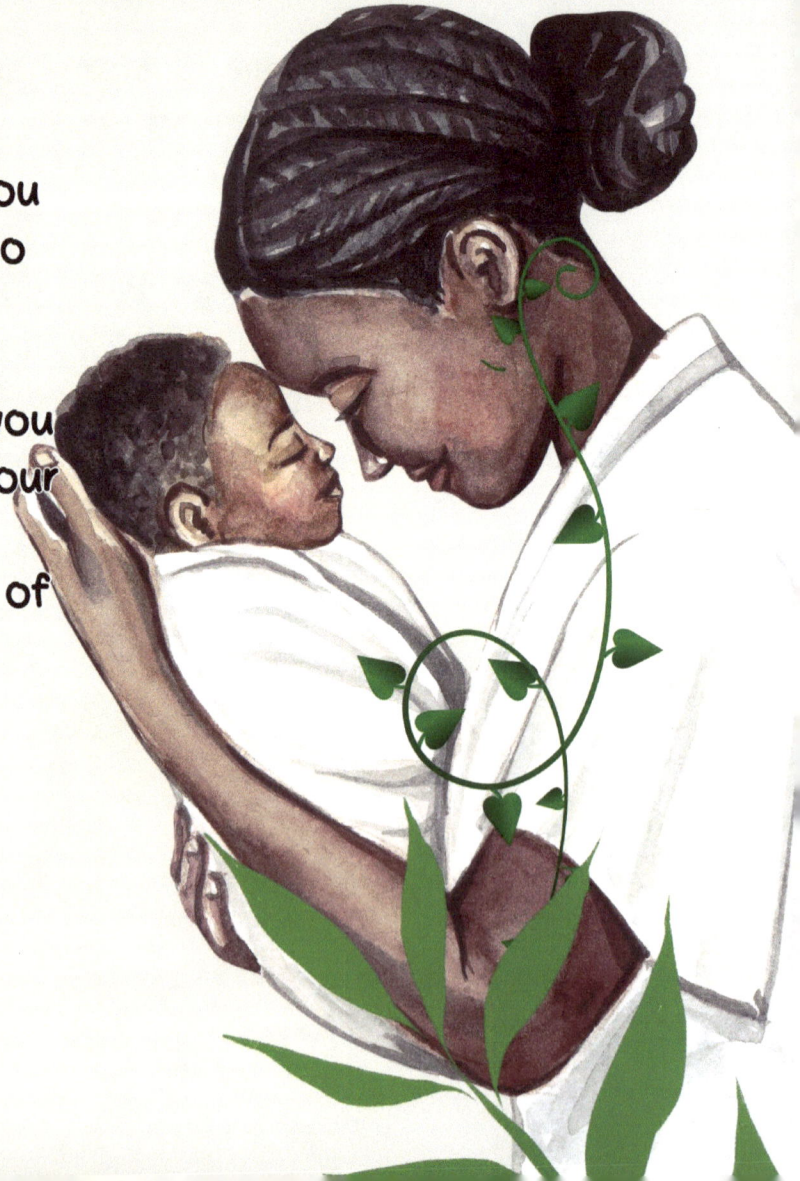

I look at you, and I fall in love each time I see you,
"So handsome, so beautiful..."
My favorite person,
So much like me and so much a part of me...
My beautiful son, even life fell in love with you.

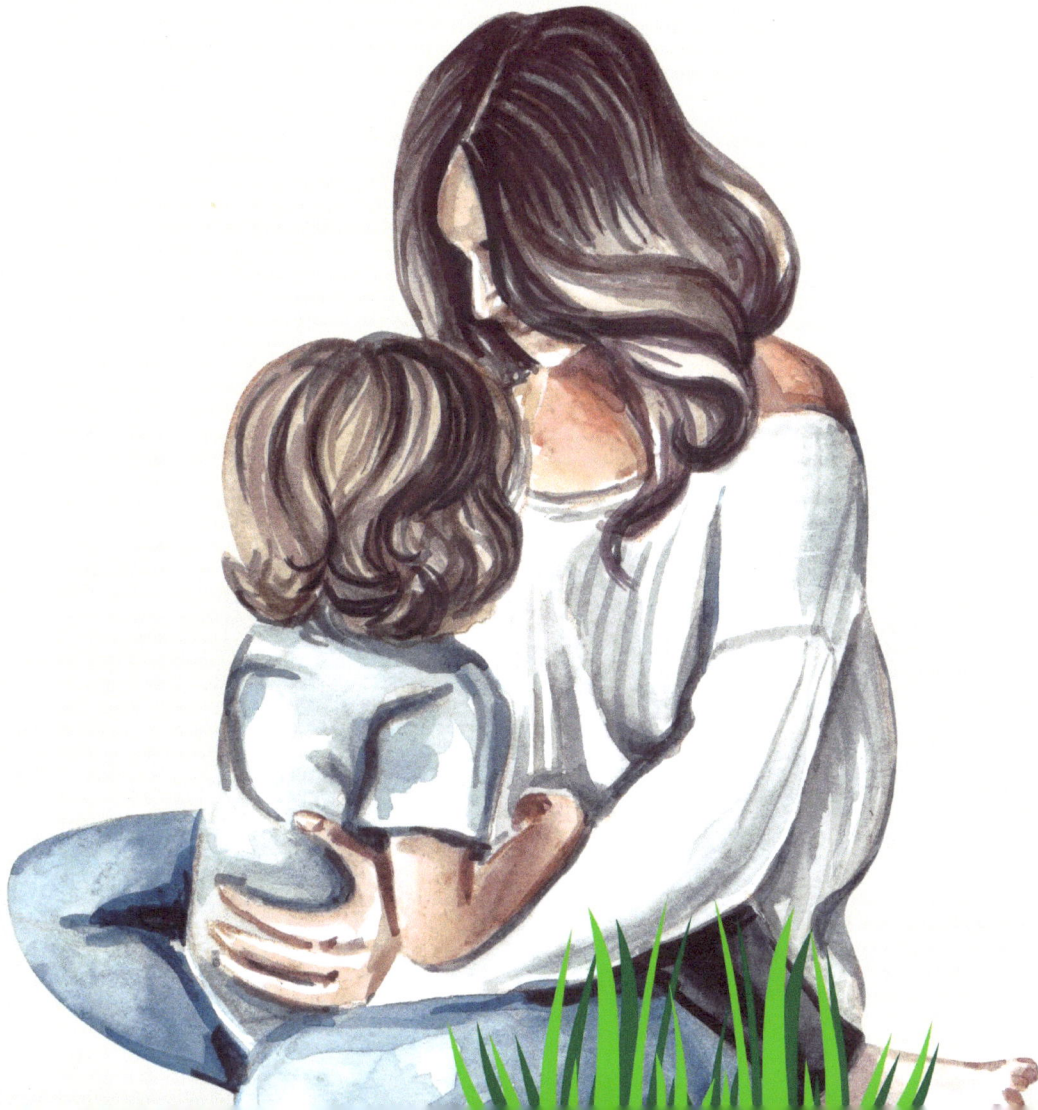

I will love you when you fail,
I will love you in your ups and
downs.
I will love your efforts,
I will always be proud of you,
even in your mistakes,
Because I know, you'll learn and
grow,
I will love you without judgment,
And there I'll be, loving you, so
strong and freely, with no
conditions,
Today I want to love you truly.

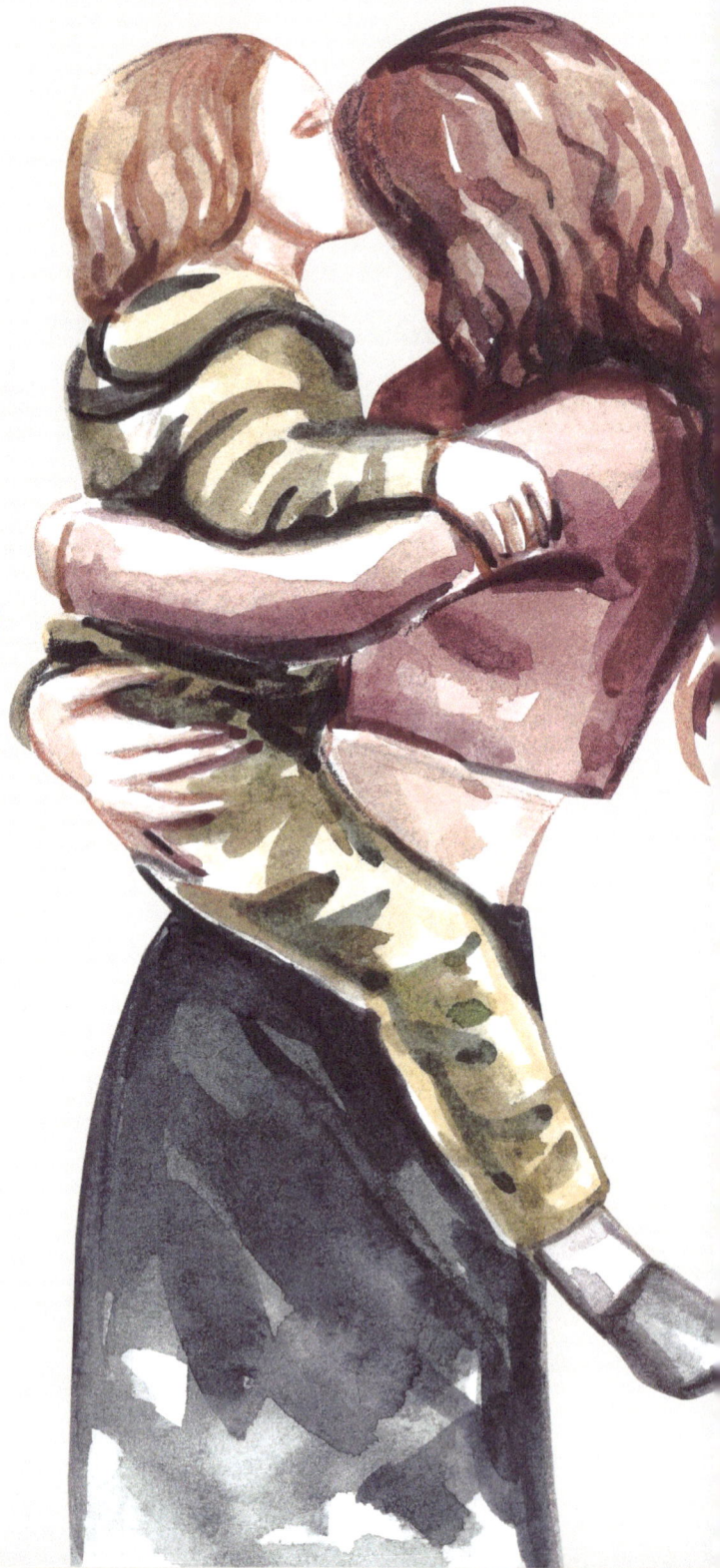

Like your smile that caresses me,
Like your presence that delights me,

I will love you again and again,
My valentine, tine, tine,
You are my valentine, tine, tine,

Because with you, every day I celebrate
my valentines.

I love you today,
and always will.

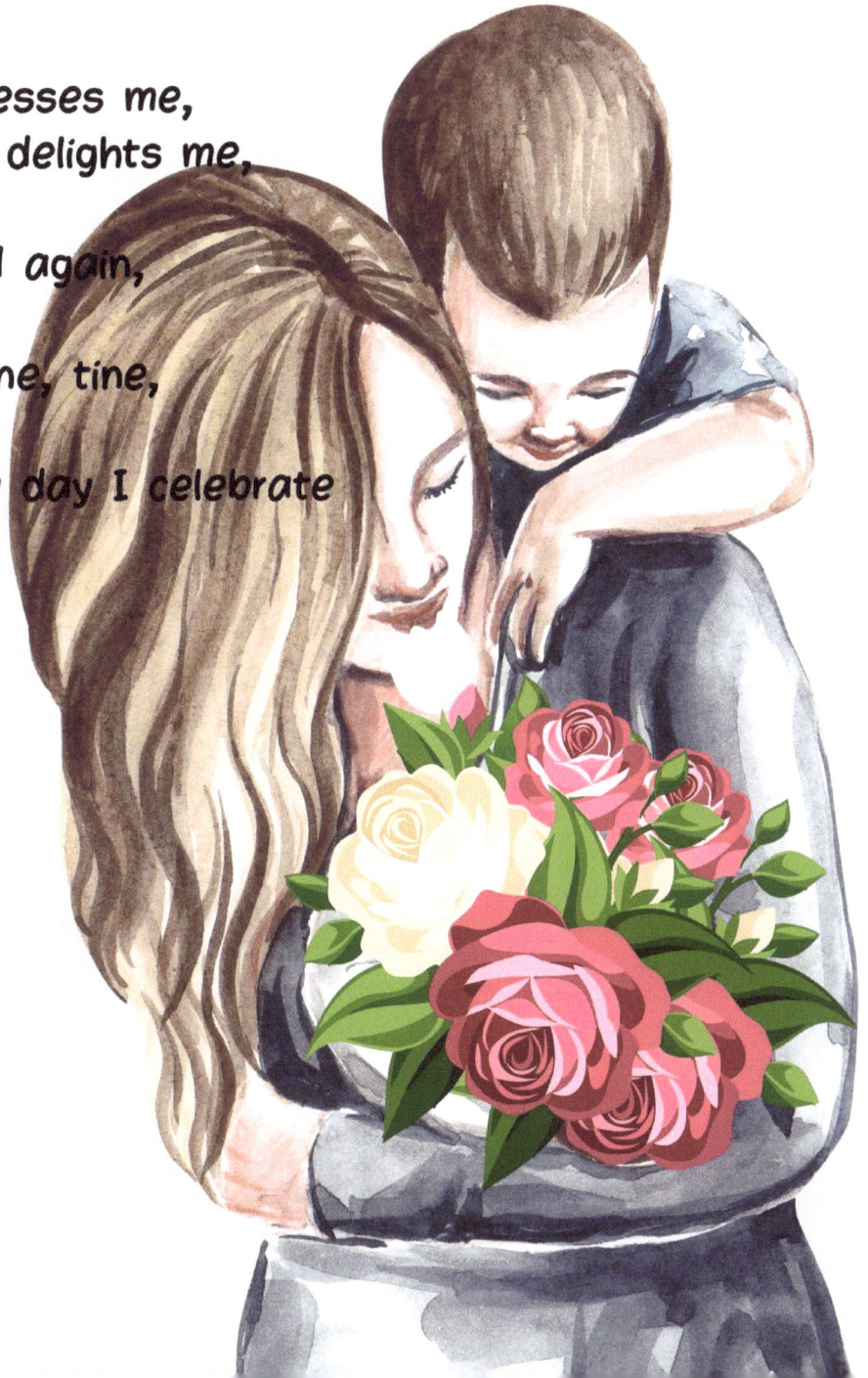

I'll bring you a trophy for every mistake
you make, and I'll say,
"It's my son trying, it's my son
succeeding and growing,

because with him there are no
mistakes, only learnings.

Because I believe in you, and I always
will. You are my hero, my
Superbubu,babo, my prince.
I love you today, and always.

My valentine, so much a part of me, so
close to me.

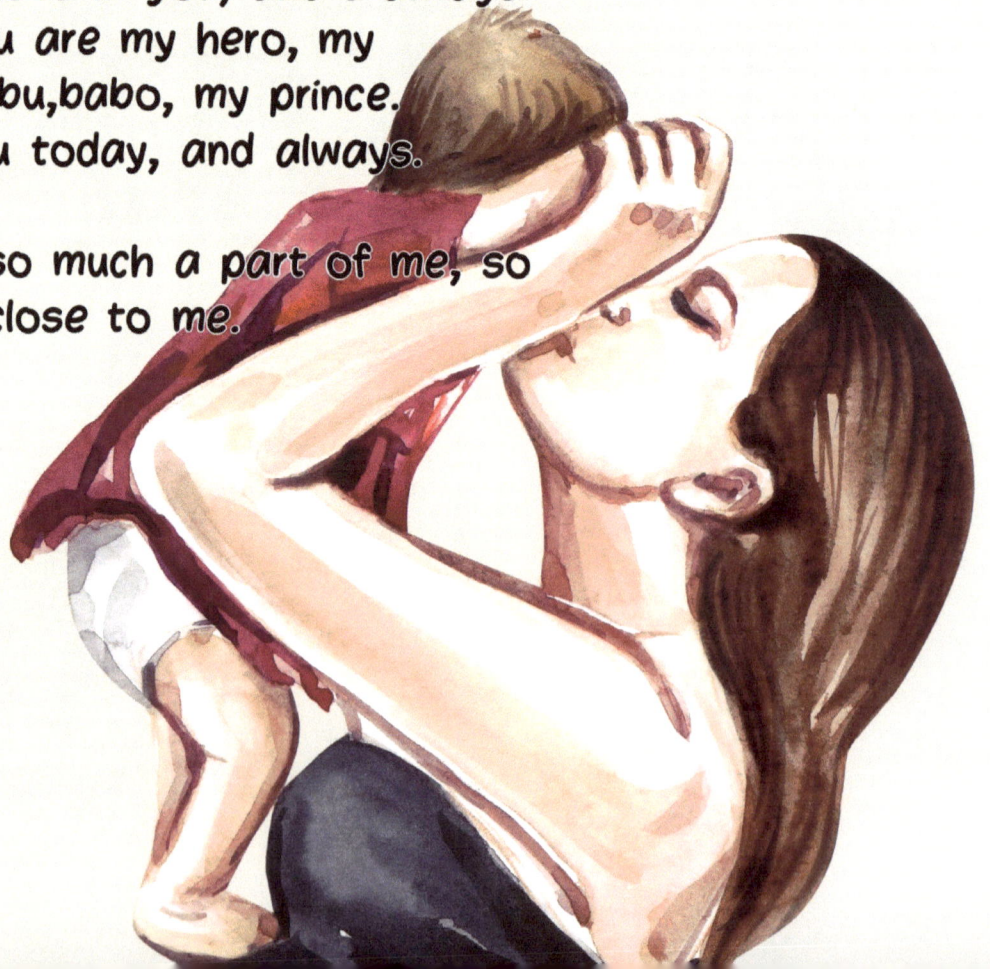

Because I know with you, I only see
the good in everything. And know
that, no matter what you do or
become, I'll always be proud of you,
simply, because you are my son.

"YOU ARE ENOUGH"

You'll always be ENOUGH for me,
my darling.

Today I love you truly, with no limits
or conditions, my baby.
You always be momma's baby.

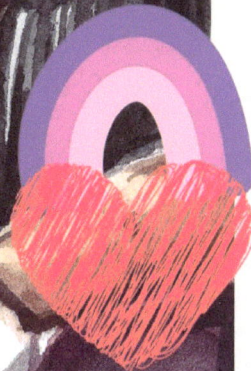

Momma will teach you, to never lose confidence in yourself,
and never doubt that you are ENOUGH,

no matter what happens or what you do. I will be always
here; loving you, strongly, telling you "You are a good son".
You are my good son.

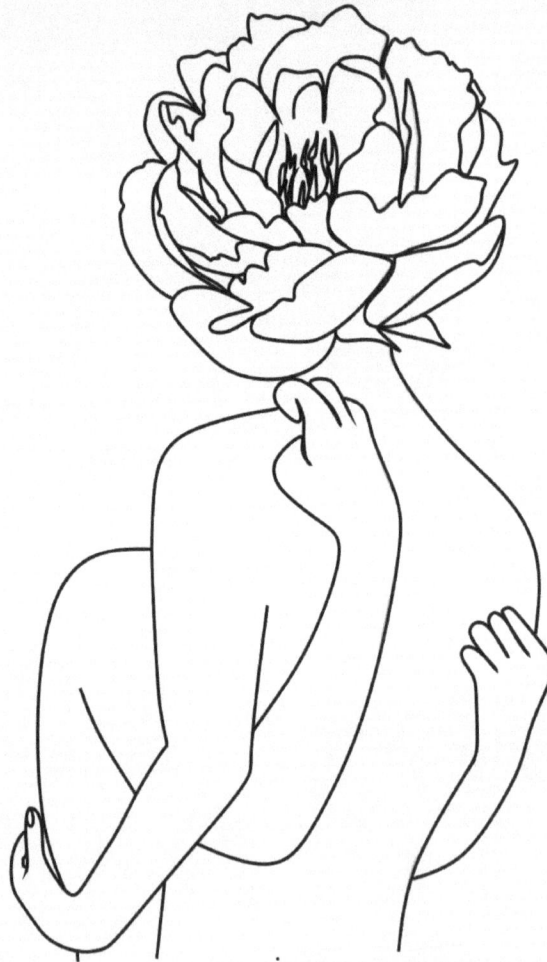

and if one day, you want to cry; my arms will always be here for you,
momma won't judge, momma will only listen, my love. Until you let it out and feel better,
my darling.

And if you fall, I will be here, to hold you up and tell you: "You can do it, my child, you can do it; trust in yourself because I trust in you.

And if one day life will take you away, I will be there waiting patiently for you, until you come back. But without judging you.
That's the promise I make to myself.

My valentine, tine, tine; I close my eyes and here you are, my Valentine, today I love you my Valentine.

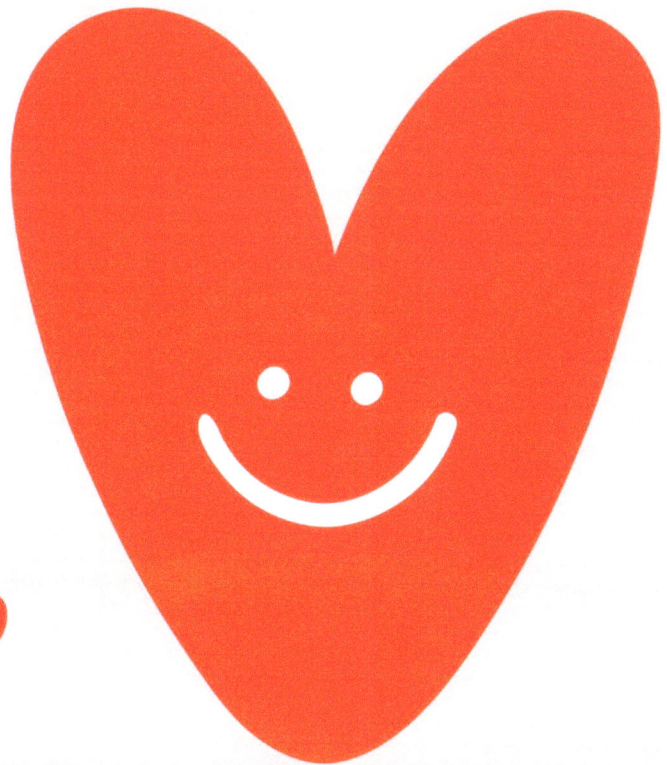

hello

I'll love you, I'll love you, I'll love you,
uncontrollably and unconditionally,
My sweet Valentine, Valentine.
You teach me how to love, my Valentine,
and If you allow me, I'll guide you on your every step.

though I know that you will be the one to guide me, in
every step I take with you.
Today I love you, and always will.

MO-MA-MA-MA

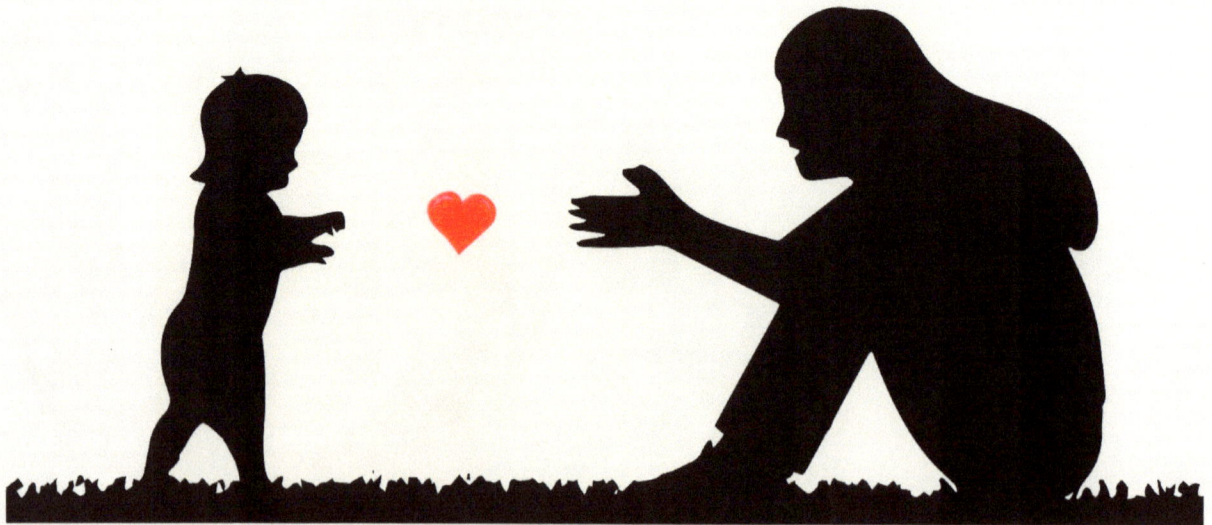

THANK YOU FOR BEING MY VALENTINE 'S DAY GIFT

Thank you for being my reason,
Today I am strong,

You are the reason why I come back home,
You are the reason why I am coming home,
You are the reason I come home,

You are my HOME, my baby,"
You are my Valentine's home, BUBU
Today I love you, and always will.
My valentine, tine, tine. Always my valentine.

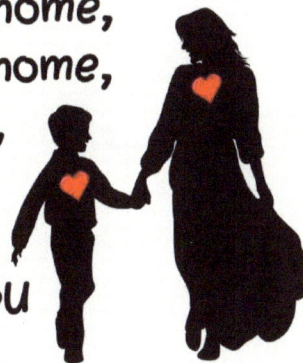

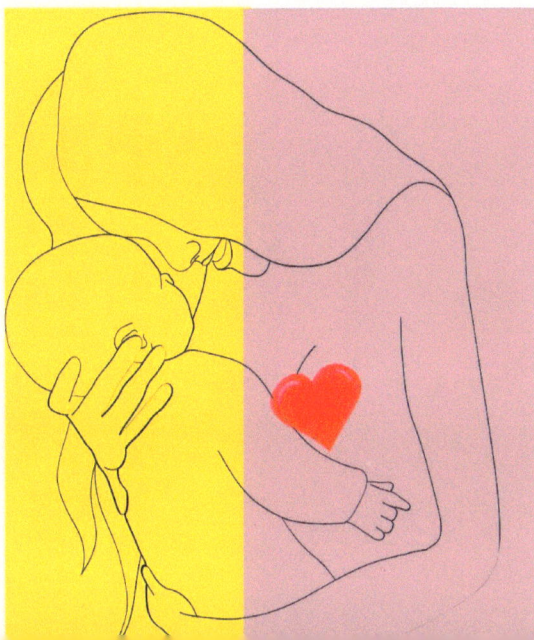

I will love you without fears, without ever
opposing your happiness,
Because I understand that true love has
no conditions or controls,

I will love you because I want to love you
truly, as God loves you, my Valentine,
tine, tine, you are my Valentine, my
darling.

"No better gif than you"

This heart belongs to
momma and son.

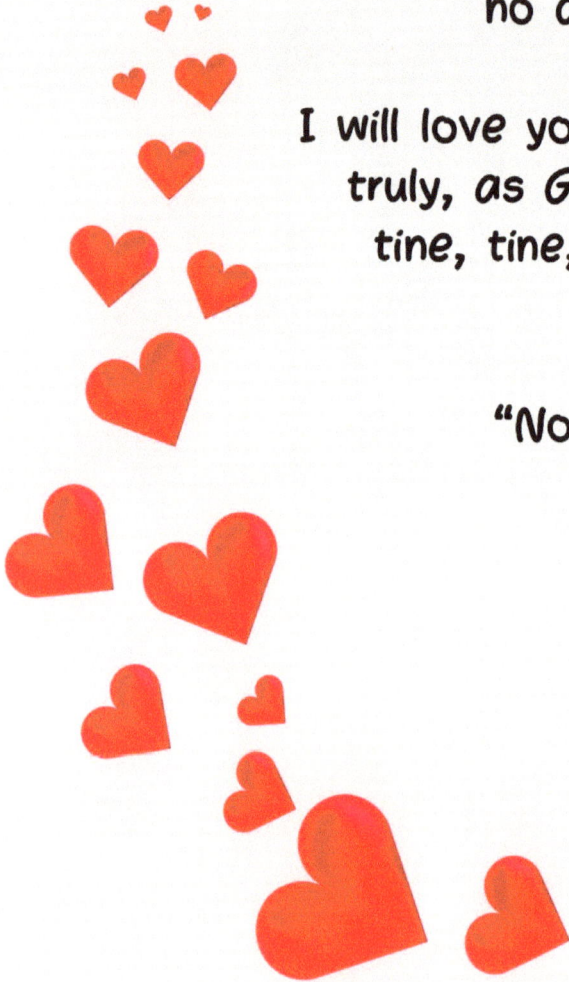

God has sent me Happiness, you, the definition of my happiness,
I love you because you are true love,
My valentine, tine, tine, you will always be my Valentine,

I will always love you, even when you have tantrums and cry, I will
be there loving you, strongly.

When you feel upset, Patiently, I will wait, for you to come and vent
in my arms, whenever you need me, if that makes you feel better.
I will be patient with you my son.
Because patience is you.

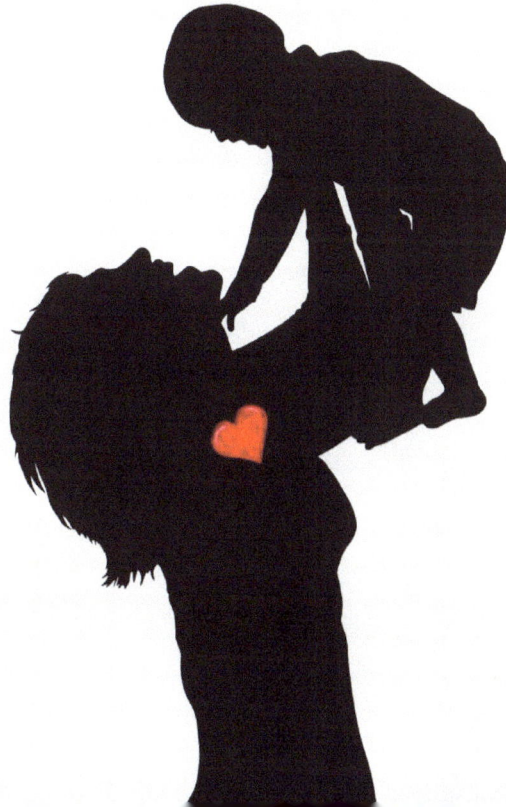

Like your smile, that lights up my life,
Like your eyes, that gives me life,
Like your existence, that brought me back to life.

Today I want to love you without limits or conditions,
Today I want to love you as God loves you,
Free and unconditionally,
My valentine, valentine, valentineeee, you will always be
my valentine, my darling.

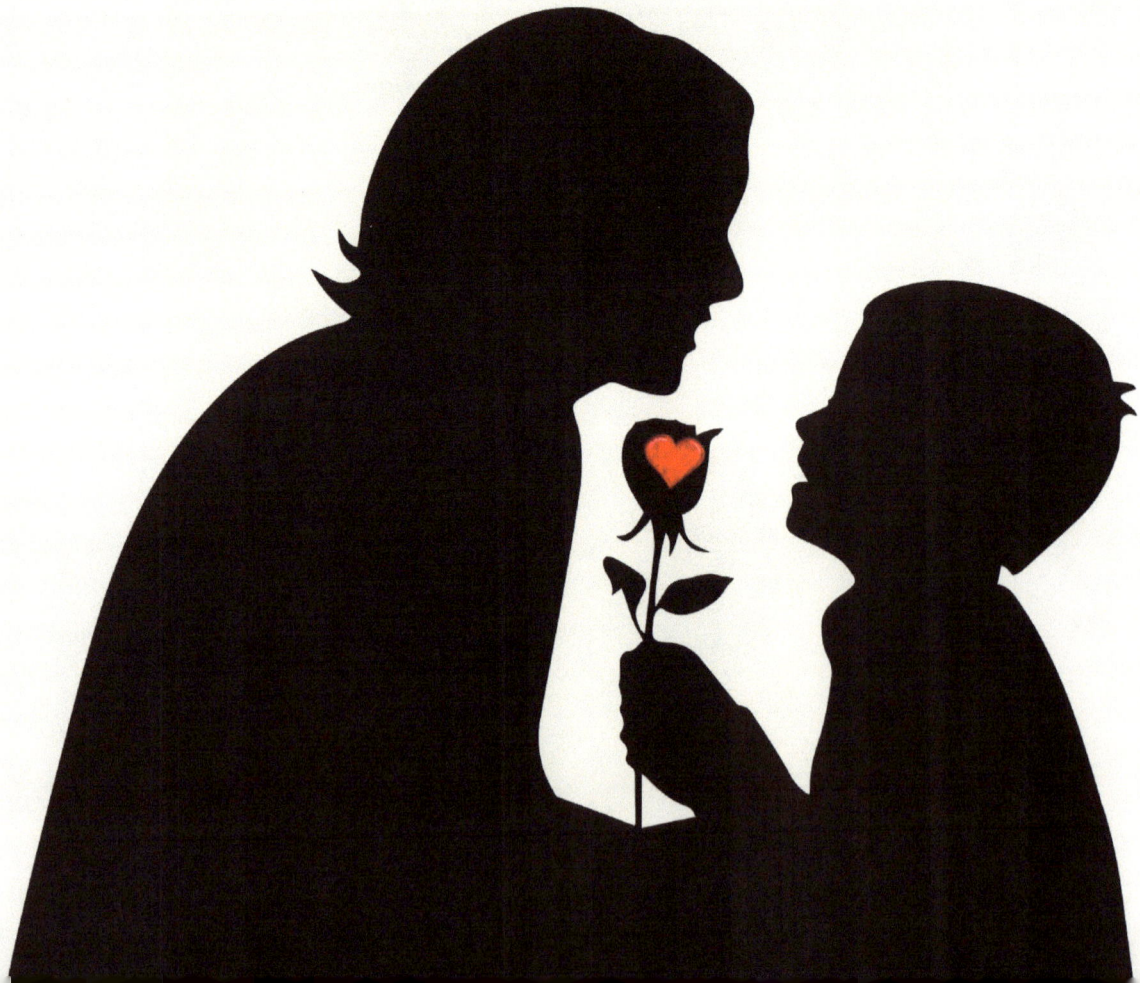

Like a rose that dresses her beauty in my garden, so are you in my eyes my child. My eyes are your Garden.

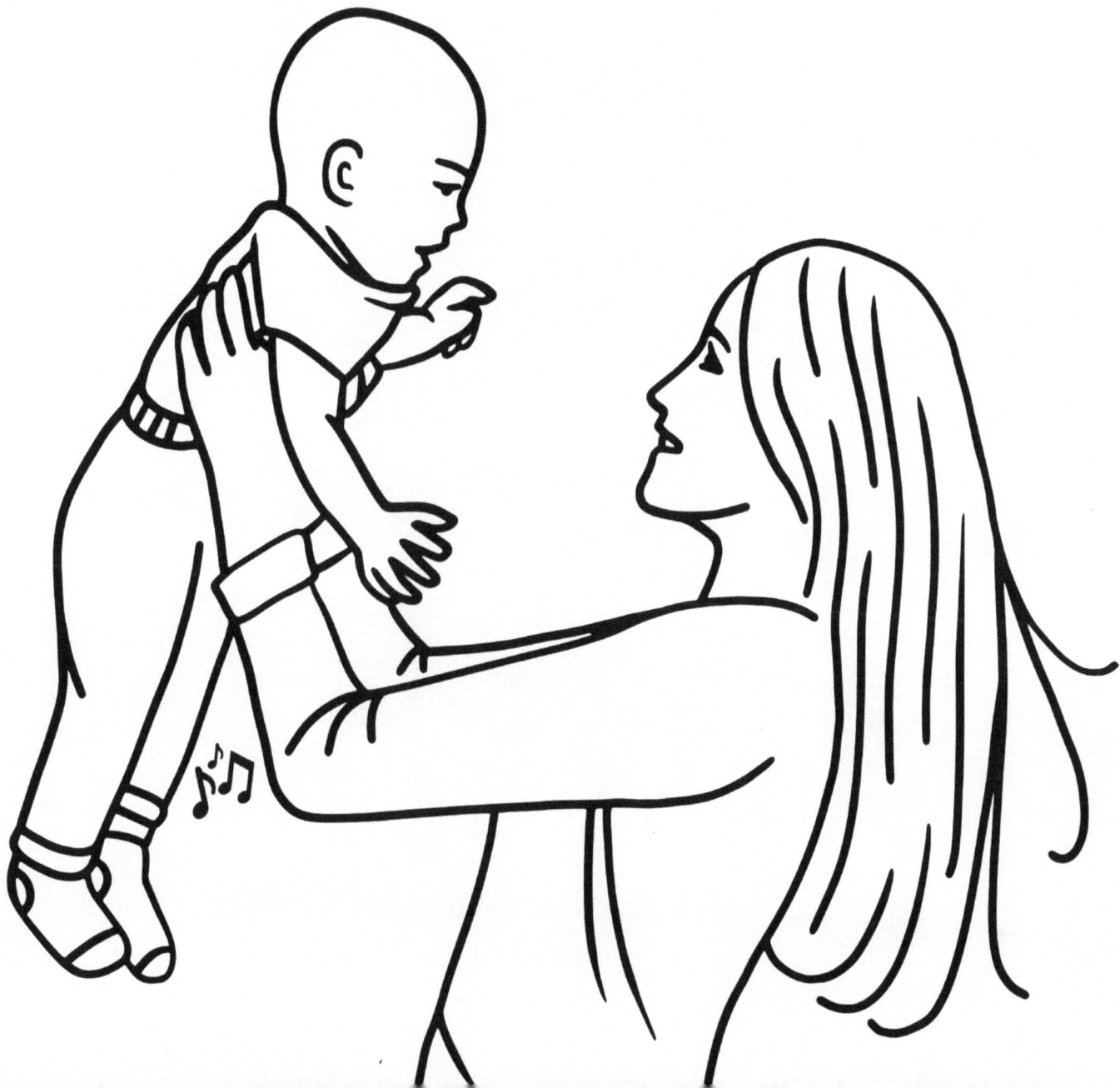

Because you share that beauty my Child. ♫

I love you, my Valentine, because you are the "bestest" thing that happened to me.

And everyone loves you, my bubu, babo; everyone.

Aunt loves you,
Grandma loves you,
Even Dodo the puppy loves you.
See?
Everybody loves you, my child,
the right people will always love you.

But that doesn't mean you have to earn love to be
loved. it happens naturally, my child.
The right people always will.
Because you deserve to be loved, my bubu, babo.

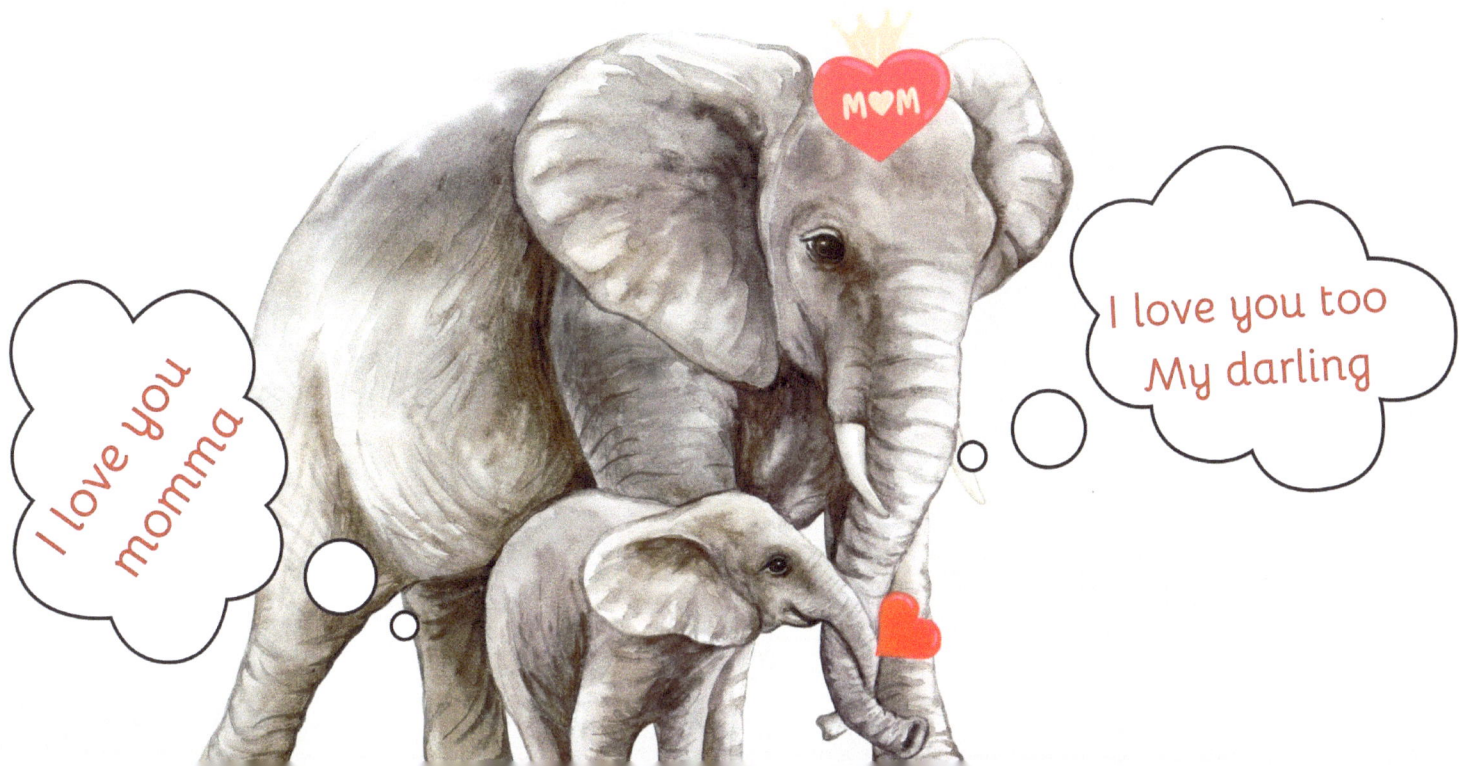

Who wouldn't love you, my darling?
If, each time I am close to you,
I Love you more,

If it's so easy to love you, my darling,
Anyone would fall in love just by looking at you,
with the beautiful smile that you illuminate,

so handsome, so beautiful,
You are the definition of love,
You are my Valentine, my darling.

I love ya, my

Valentine

The right people will always love you., love you, love you, my baby,
But who wouldn't love you, my bubu, babo?

Auntie brought you chocolates,
Grandpa brought you flowers,
And Dodo wagged her little tail to welcome you,
And let's not forget Uncle Tom, who sang to you,
the Valentine's song.

He is so happy to be a first-time uncle, Tom.
See? Everybody loves you, my baby,
The whole family adores you,

Because loving you is as easy as breathing,
And me? I love you more than life itself,
You have my whole heart, my baby,
Today, and always, my heart is yours.
Thank you for being my valentines, today.

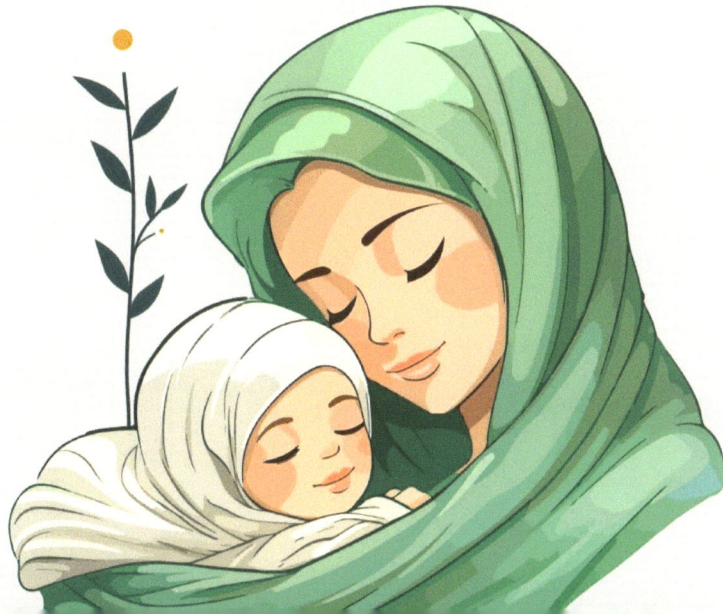

When I am close to you, it feels like home,
"You are my home, my baby,"
You are my Valentine 's home,

I feel so good being close to you, my baby.
I love you so much.

_So much?
So, so, so, much.

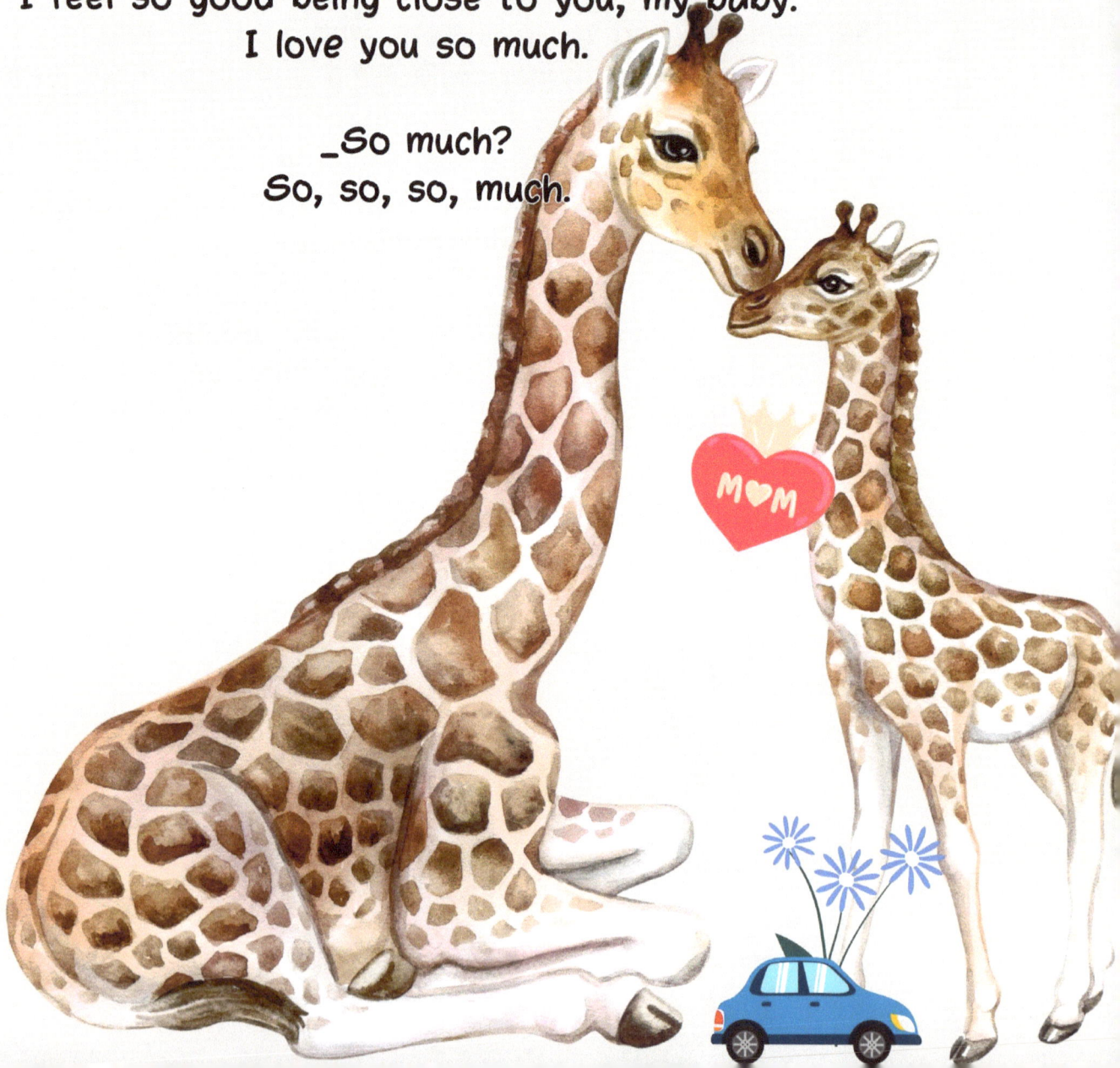

You are the reason why I come back home,
You are the reason why I am coming home,
You are the reason I come home,

You my baby, you are my home,
My Valentine's home. I like you so much.

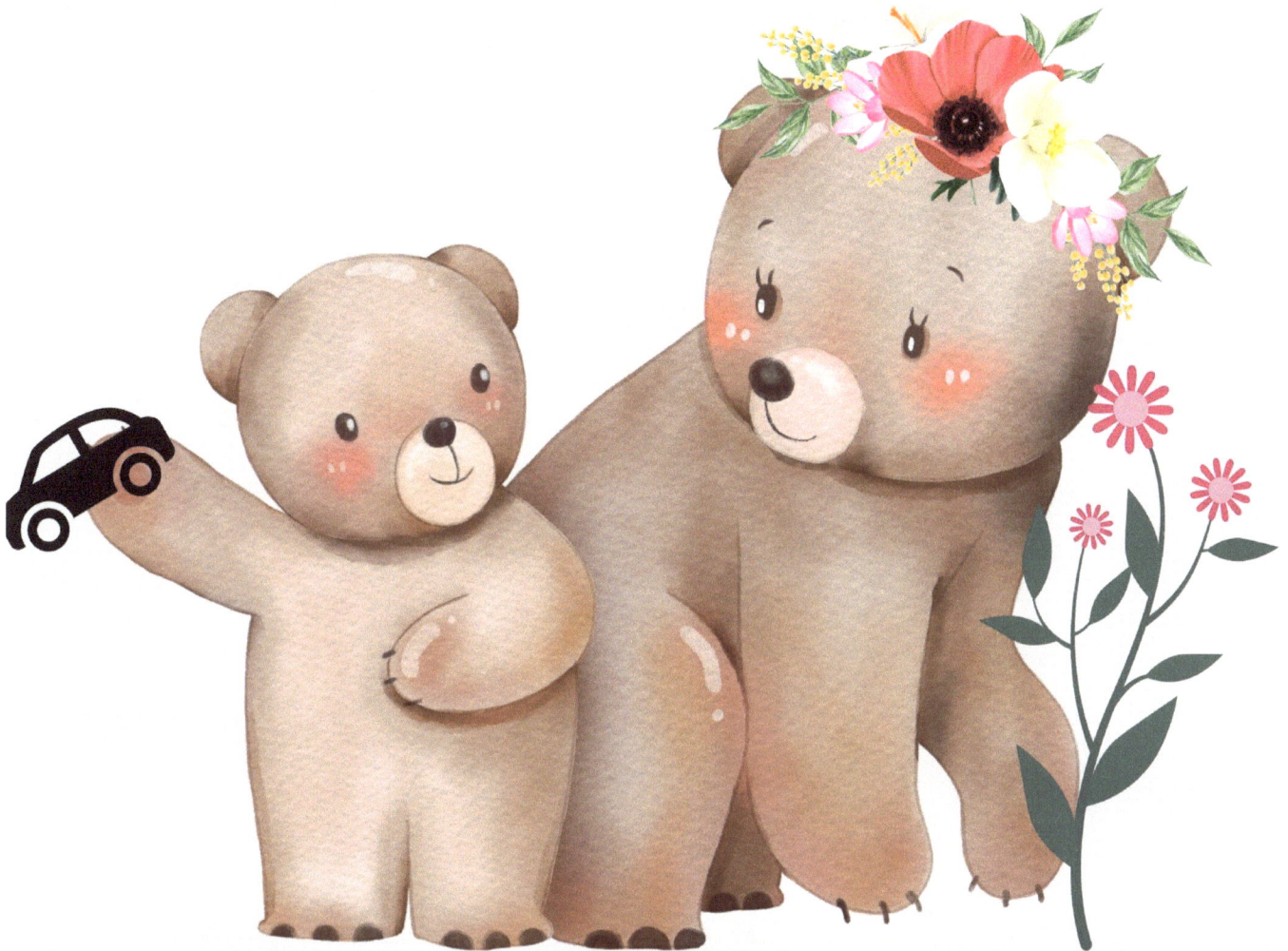

Each time, when I look at you, I melt in your presence,
because each time, I am close to you, I know more, what love is

Each time, when I am near to you, just amazing words come to me,
it is, the first time, my feelings have found words.

You are my poetry; you are my love.
with you, I can explain what I feel. with you everything is easy.

Today I feel strong.
Today I love, and always will.

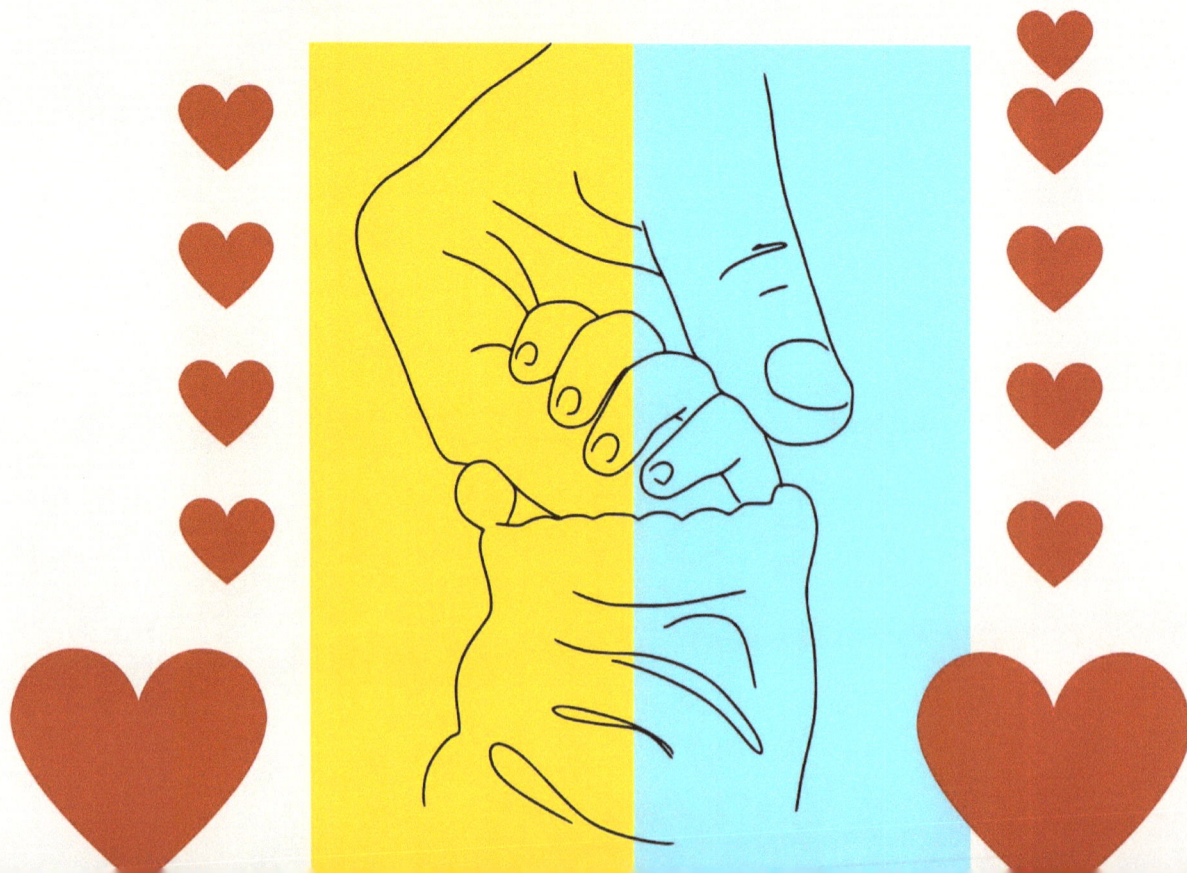

I hug you, and
It feels always GOOD being close to you.
You are my "home," my baby,
You are the definition of 'love."
My valentine, tine, tine,tine,
You are my valentine, my bubu, babo.

I love you today, and always will, my darling.
You are my son forever, my bubuuuu.
And I always be your mo-ma-ma.

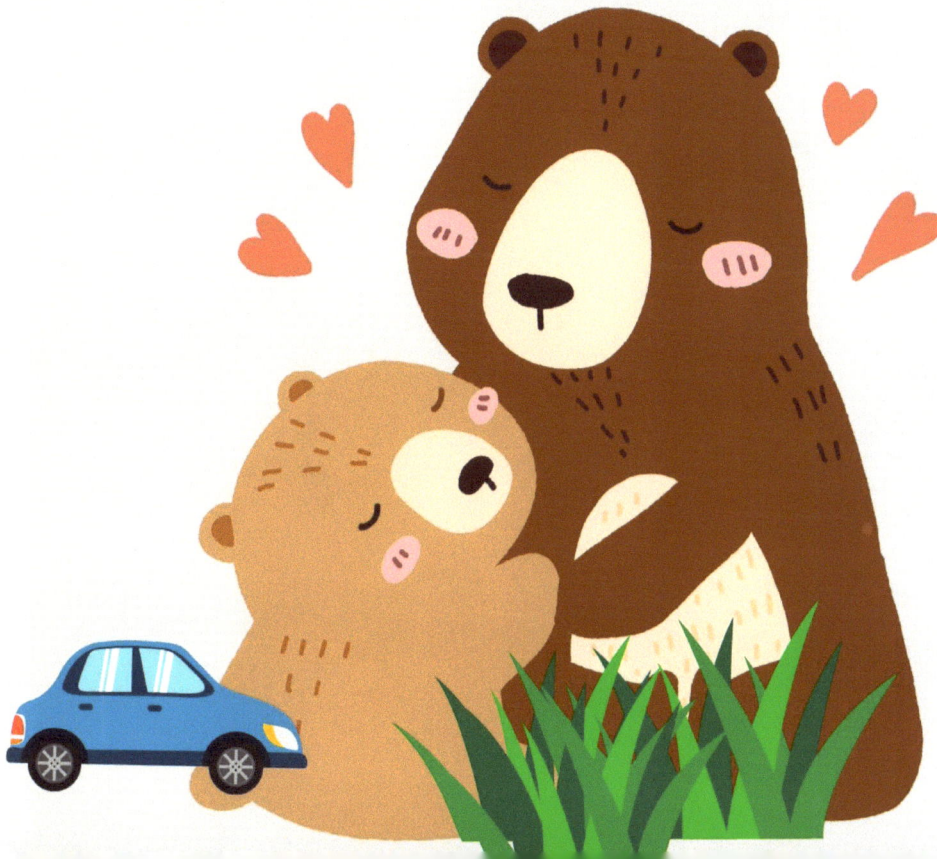

I will love you without barriers,
I will love you without limits,
I will love you so much; until one day "You'll love
your baby just as much, if that's what you choose."
And you'll remember the way momma loved you,
because you will always be momma's baby, no
matter how time passes. I will always love you, my
darling

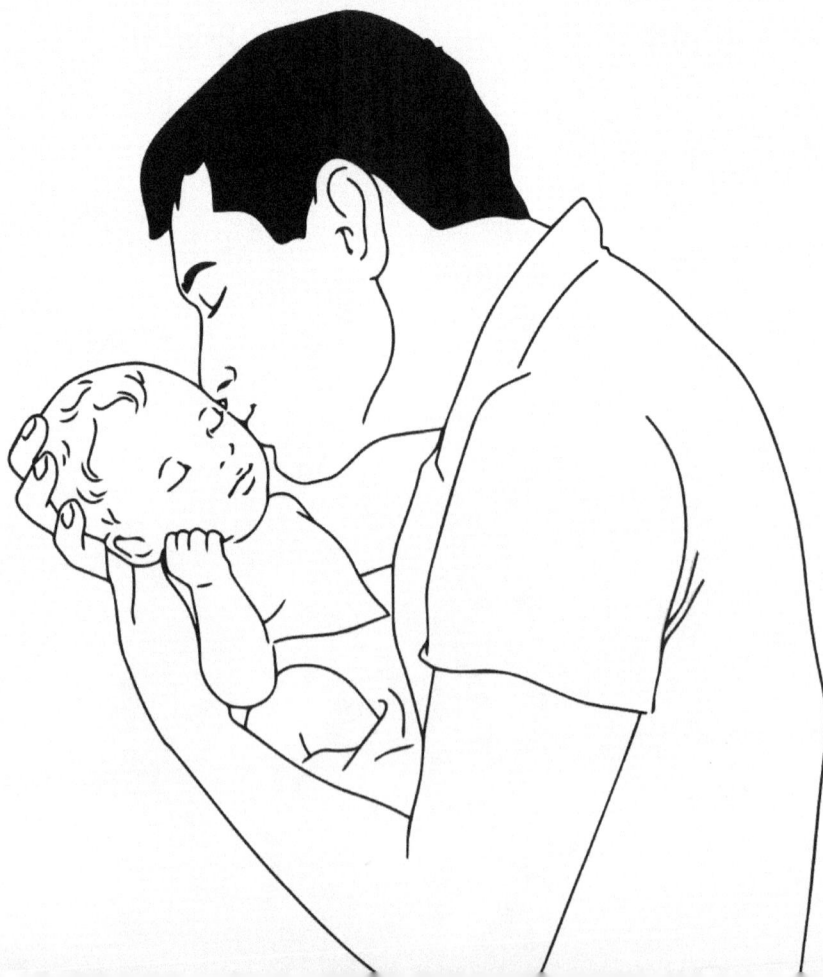

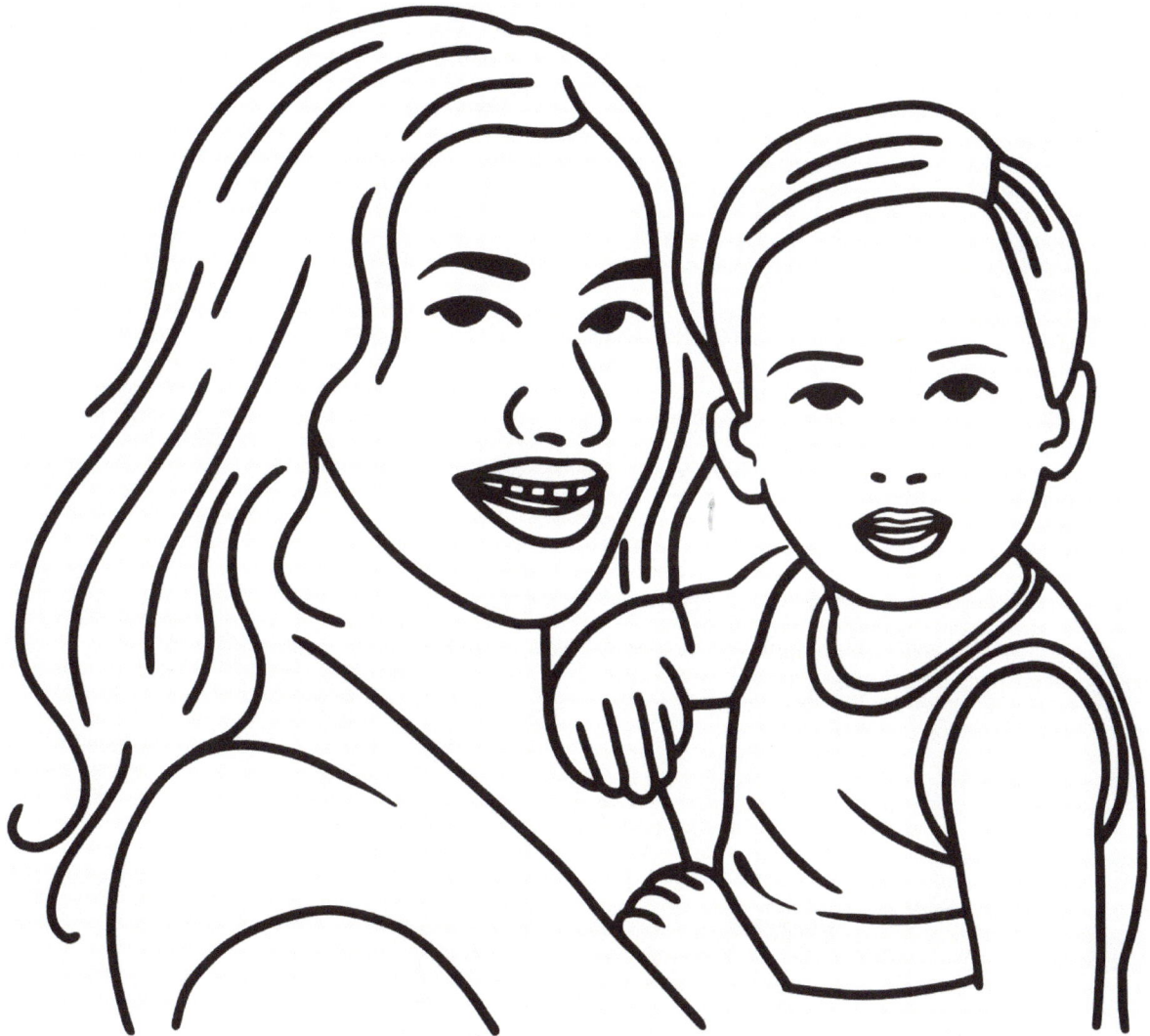

Thank you ❤️

REVIEW

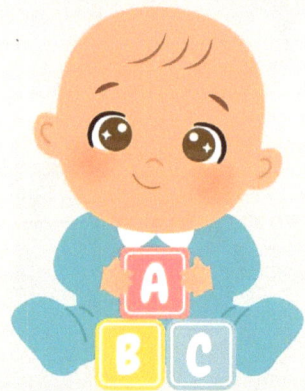

"Happy Love's Day "

Dear reader, this is another fantastic book, adding to the wealth of mesmerizing works out there, where EVERYONE stands on their UNIQUE essence and purity.
I want to "thank you" personally for your support to me, and all the authors.
"Our first Valentine's Day", for me, is a world of love" I hope you and your baby have had many deep moments of connection and love.
I dedicate this "son- poem" to you because I made it from my heart.

As an author, comments from readers like you open doors for others to enjoy a laugh as well. Feedback not only helps me improve as a writer but also helps other readers discover the book and benefit as human beings from this creativity or even decide if it's right for them.

To SHARE YOUR EXPERIENCE IN A REVIEW on Amazon, just go to the book page and click on the "Write a customer review" button. I would love to hear your thoughts on the book and would appreciate any feedback.
Thank you again for your support and for choosing to share this journey with me.
I hope you enjoyed the book, and I look forward to hearing from you soon.

Instagram @angelicarockford -The author
Twitter & Instagram @sunkullaybooks -The brand (sunkullay and angelica Rockford)
TikTok @angelicarockford @sunkullay
Facebook @sunkullay & Angelica Rockford.

Acknowledgment.

"I would like to express my heartfelt gratitude to the talented singers from Peru, such as William Luna, Los Shapis, Los Apus, Gian Marco, Susana Baca, Luis Pacheco, and Max Castro, among many others. Their incredible artistry has been a source of inspiration for me since childhood. Their music has touched my soul and played a significant role in shaping my own work. And lastly, to my sister and my own experiences(life). I am forever grateful for the passion and creativity they have brought into the world, which continues to inspire me on my own artistic journey."

www.ingramcontent.com/pod-product-compliance
Lightning Source LLC
Chambersburg PA
CBHW041240020426
42333CB00002B/31

9 781738 230723